T0160828

WHEN FORCE MEETS FATE

A MISSION TO SOLVE
AN INVISIBLE ILLNESS

JAMISON HILL

Copyright © 2020 Jamison Hill
All rights reserved.

No part of this book may be reproduced, or stored in a retrieval system,
or transmitted in any form or by any means, electronic, mechanical,
photocopying, recording, or otherwise, without express written permission
of the publisher.

Published by Inkshares, Inc., Oakland, California
www.inkshares.com

Edited by Avalon Radys & Sarah Nivala
Cover design by Tim Barber
Interior design by Kevin G. Summers

ISBN: 9781950301157
e-ISBN: 9781950301164
Library of Congress Control Number: 2020945547

First edition

Printed in the United States of America

AUTHOR'S NOTE

I relied on my memory, personal journal, and blog posts to write this book. I also used audio recordings and interviews to corroborate events and reconstruct dialogue, which may not always be verbatim. In recounting the car accident, I referenced articles and the official accident report from the California Highway Patrol. Nine names have been changed in the book—one doctor, one cat, and seven others. The rest are real, as are all of their identifying traits. Some of the dates and times are condensed and approximate. For more, see the complete author's note in the back of the book.

FOREWORD

My life as a freelance writer was pure hustle in 2016. I worked after my daughters were asleep and whenever I could during the day, often with my youngest sleeping on my lap. One week I added it up, and I had worked sixty hours—twenty of which were dedicated to ME/CFS (myalgic encephalomyelitis/chronic fatigue syndrome).

The multisystem disease was slowly killing an old friend of mine, Whitney Dafoe, who had been featured in *Forgotten Plague,* a documentary about ME/CFS. I reached out to Ryan Prior, the film's codirector, and became a board member and later an employee of his nonprofit, the Blue Ribbon Foundation.

When I suggested creating a "Share Your Story" page for the foundation's website, I thought it'd be a good way for people with ME/CFS to talk about their experiences. Dozens of stories poured in from patients who wanted to share their struggles, and I read them with increasing heartache. After I edited and posted them online, the stories were shared rapidly throughout the ME/CFS community. Then one came in from Jamison Hill.

"It's afternoon, about two o'clock, and I just woke up for the second time today," he wrote.

Jamison also had been featured in *Forgotten Plague*. In the film, Jamison laughs often, his dimples deepening into his cheeks, his bright blue eyes shining despite being one of the millions missing out on a healthy life because of ME/CFS.

It's been nearly a decade since Jamison went from living a life of an active twenty-two-year-old college student to lying severely ill in a hospital bed. His story is one of the terrifying ones: he went to the gym one morning like he always did, but suddenly he became too weak to walk, and he hasn't been the same since.

Before Jamison submitted his story for me to publish, I'd only heard that he'd become one of the most severe cases of ME/CFS. I'd seen GoFundMe fundraisers to help with his housing, medical expenses, and treatment. When Ryan spoke of him, his voice grew soft, a tone I'd come to recognize in the ME/CFS community as being reserved for a person who'd taken a turn for the worse. A person who was living a form of death.

Jamison later explained that he'd been stuck in a cave for the last eighteen months, unable to speak or chew food. Coming out of it thanks to experimental treatments was a rebirth for him. Even though he had a chance at a new life, he was still unable to walk or sit up in bed on his own. But suddenly he could make sounds that people understood; sometimes he could even speak full sentences. He could eat food. He could communicate with people through email and text. His story was one of hope.

"I can sit at a forty-five degree angle and speak polysyllabic words, sometimes even short sentences," he wrote, "and people can actually hear me. It's wonderful. To go from silent to audible is an invigorating, albeit humbling, experience."

After I published his story, we started emailing each other, then texting. It was late-July, and I'd just gotten my first book deal. Jamison was working on his memoir, and I fumbled through helping him get some of his essays published. By mid-November, I brought my daughter, Mia, with me to meet him in person.

We flew to San Francisco, where I picked up a car I'd rented, then drove to Palo Alto to the home where Whitney's parents, Janet and Ron, had been caring for Whitney for a decade. This was my second visit that year. I knew he would be too ill to see me, but the visit was worth it to spend time with his family, who felt like my extended family.

A large part of that trip's purpose was to see Jamison. I drove three hours east through California's Central Valley with Mia, Janet, and Ashley, Whitney's sister, so we could visit with Jamison and his mom, Kathleen. Jamison and I had sent messages beforehand, excited to finally see each other.

When we arrived, Kathleen welcomed us. She'd prepared dinner, and whenever she mentioned Jamison, she made a motion with her head to a room down the hall. Before we all sat down to eat a regular meal, she mixed up a smoothie in a large cup with a straw for her son, smiling as she did. I wondered how it had been for her when Jamison had been at his worst, unable to eat. I looked over at Mia, who had refused to eat the vegetables on her plate, but I couldn't imagine the desperation in not being able to feed her at all.

Before entering Jamison's room, I was worried what germs I might have on my clothes. A simple cold or virus could knock him down further. I was worried that seeing me would cause him to crash. But mainly I was worried that he'd go beyond his limits and wake up the next morning feeling horrible and unable to move. So we smiled at each other. I hugged him a bunch and held his hand. We made jokes, told a few dating horror stories, and then it was time for us to give him a break.

We texted late into the night. I kept asking him if he felt all right. He said yes and that he wanted to see us again. I bought him some tea from his favorite little shop the following afternoon, and some fudge. We drove up to his house as the sun was setting and took some pictures on the porch. I went inside to use the bathroom, then snuck across the hall to Jamison's room.

He had thick blankets on the windows and the lights off. I couldn't see anything, until I saw the faint light from his phone—his signal to tell me where he was. I saw his shape then. He wasn't sitting up. He was on his left side, bent over almost in a fetal position, his cheek pressed against the bed. Crashed.

I felt his hand reach out for mine and sank to my knees at the same time. My other arm went around his back, my right cheek on his head. He only had boxers on with a sheet covering his legs and feet. Kathleen came in to uncover the windows so we could see each other. I stayed that way for a bit, whispering that he should have told me that he had what ME/CFS patients call "the world's worst hangover."

He wanted to know how long we were staying, where we were going next, and, of course, he offered ideas of where to eat dinner. He couldn't talk like he had the day before. Most of the communication I either figured out through pantomime, or he had to type out on his phone.

After everyone else had a chance to visit with him, I went in to see Jamison a second time. I kneeled by his bed to say goodbye. He held my hand tight and whispered, "I'm so tired of this shit."

I told him that he was constantly in my thoughts. That I loved him. And that I'd miss him dearly. That I'd be back to visit as soon as I could, to be there more than just an hour or two. "I'll spoon you next time," I said, and he chuckled.

I stood out in the living room, watching Janet hug Kathleen. "We have amazing sons," Janet said.

They were crying—a stark contrast to the night before, when we'd been celebrating Jamison's recovery. Kathleen went in to check on Jamison and said he wanted us all to come back, stand in the hallway, and wave goodbye one more time.

"He just wants to see your faces again," Kathleen said. We stood there, blowing kisses, waving, watching him do it in return from his dark room. The cave.

The next day, as I told him I was on my way to the airport, he sent me a text: "Damn. Don't go."

From the moment I'd left the hallway of his room, I hadn't wanted to. It's a different sort of grief, to feel too helpless, too far away, and isolated.

When I later read what Jamison wrote on his blog about our visit, what stuck out most to me was that he'd hoped his recovery, however incomplete, would give us hope. Jamison wished that seeing him—smiling and sitting up—would give us, his largest group of visitors in years, new hope for Whitney to recover.

But Jamison's just like that. He's easily one of the happiest, lovable humans I know. In the years that we've been emailing and texting back and forth, he's gone into frustrated rants maybe twice. And I usually have to specifically ask for them. Seeing him sitting there, knowing he hadn't gotten out of bed in almost two years, I was completely in awe of his ability to maintain any semblance of who he'd been years earlier.

When I returned home that evening, I gave a reading to a class of about forty students. I stood at a podium and held a printed copy of the essay I'd recently had published about Whitney.

"This piece is really raw for me right now," I said.

Every time I looked up, I saw blank faces, mouths agape, and one student was audibly crying. When I finished, I opened the floor to questions, and there was nothing but silence. Then the girl who had been crying raised her hand and said, "Is your friend okay?"

I took a deep breath and told her I'd just been at his house, tried to explain what that experience had been like, then added that I'd also met Jamison, who'd been just as bad as Whitney, but he'd gotten well enough to visit with people. She smiled at that, and I did, too, because Jamison was already accomplishing his mission to bring hope.

One of the students asked me if I had any advice on writing. I told the student what everyone says: to sit in a chair and fucking write. But then I thought about Jamison, who reminds me almost daily of the sheer passion it takes, the absolutely necessary part that needs to exist before that.

He writes everything on his phone. He can't use a laptop, can't handle looking at the brightness of the screen. He wrote part of this book looking at his phone through tanning goggles. That amount of passion, that desire to write words, humbles me. I wrote a book from my kitchen table in low-income housing, where I parented my two daughters alone, and I deeply admire Jamison's amount of "must" to write. To live.

—*Stephanie Land*

*I never stop being amazed by
how simultaneously cruel and beautiful
this world can be.*
—Nina Riggs

PROLOGUE

The Life I Loved

I loved my life. It was hectic at times, but I relished in the discipline it took to work two jobs, attend college classes, pose for modeling gigs, and most importantly, work out every day. Exercise was my fun, my playtime—the chance for me to drown out everything and get wild. But I also saw it as my path to fame and fortune. Surely one day I would be a famous fitness personality on the cover of every muscle magazine.

I became obsessed with working out. I'd skip class and my other commitments, even go without adequate food or sleep, but I never missed a workout. While my friends were off studying in the library or partying at nightclubs, I was at the gym, my clothes drenched in sweat. Exercise was so embedded in my life, so ingrained in my daily routine, it was like breathing. I couldn't live without it.

Most days I woke up at five in the morning, downed a protein shake and caffeine pill, then at six thirty, I led a class of exercisers in an hour-long, heart-pumping, sweat-inducing, high-intensity anaerobic workout routine. When the class was finished, the floor was covered with sweat and exhausted bodies. But my day was just beginning.

From there, I went to Sonoma State University, where I spent the next several hours sitting through lectures. An average student, I did just enough to pass my courses, and if I had an opportunity, I snuck in a nap in the back of the lecture hall. When my academic classes were done, the real fun began. I'd hit the gym for three hours of heavy weightlifting, tossing ninety-pound dumbbells around the weight room as if they were pillows. And I'd finish the workout ready to take on the next challenge of my day.

Then I'd down a second protein shake and caffeine pill as I raced off to teach another group fitness class in the evening. I'd finish the class, and on my way home, make a final stop at the gym for an hour of high-intensity interval training on the treadmill. Finally, after all the calories were burned and all the sweat had hit the floor, I chugged one last protein shake and tried to sleep a few hours before I woke up and did it all over again.

Now, nine years later, my life is very different. I often try but fail to wrap my head around the stark contrast—the fact that I've tried, really tried, to walk on my own, but every time I put my feet on the ground, my muscles give out at the slightest bearing of weight. I used to lift hundreds of pounds, now I'm too weak to hold a water glass, and I have to type these words on a smartphone because my laptop is too heavy.

But these are just some of the obstacles I've encountered. I was in a traumatic car accident that left me haunted by sinister images of broken windshields and burning bodies. Then, a year and a half later, I contracted myalgic encephalomyelitis, the disease that has stolen my ability to walk, talk, and eat solid food.

I've witnessed my health steadily crumble over the last decade, but it's still hard for me to imagine how a fit, active, seemingly healthy person in the prime of life can be reduced to such profound debilitation. Perhaps that's why I can't seem to reconcile my past self with my present self, why I'm still waiting to get my life back, still waiting to wake up tomorrow and resume everything that I was doing before I got sick.

I can't help but wonder whether I'm any semblance of the person I used to be—the same person who was healthy enough to go on road trips and see movies with friends, the same person who loved life so intensely that sleep was an inconvenience, the same person who cared about working out more than anything else, the same person who used to throw weights around the gym, then wake up at five in the morning to teach group fitness classes. *Am I still that person? Do I even want to be that person anymore?*

These questions are hard to ask, and even harder to answer, but they've shown me a lot about myself and the obstacles I've faced. As much as I wish I could've steered my fate away from the obstacles in my path, I can't ignore the fact that they've made me who I am. It's because of them that I became a writer. This book only exists because I lived through a tragic car accident and a devastating illness. These obstacles have made me wiser and more self-aware. They've shown me the wisdom of my mortality, that nobody is invincible, not even a young, healthy person who works out every day.

I also can't ignore that the obstacles were always waiting on the horizon, as is any potential danger, but like an inexperienced pilot flying low over foggy terrain, I hadn't yet learned how to avoid them. Then, before I knew it, they were right in front of me and I had no choice but to crash head-on.

YEAR 0

Coping With Trauma

CHAPTER 1

The Crash

June 13, 2009

The wind on the Napa River Bridge feels like thumbtacks poking my face. I lean over the side and peer down at the current slowly flowing under me, my arms clinging to the railing like a child on an inner tube floating in the water below. The water is calm and peaceful, the opposite of how I feel inside.

My body surges with adrenaline, as if I just chugged five cups of coffee. All I can think about is what it would feel like to jump—maybe nothing, maybe everything; maybe, just for a second, it would feel like drifting through outer space. It's a thought as scary as it sounds and one I shouldn't entertain for long because surviving such a fall—like the kid who jumped head-first off the Golden Gate Bridge and broke his back—would be the most agonizing experience of my life. That is, except for what has just happened.

I turn away from the water and the thumbtacks, my blurry vision darting across the concrete shoulder, and then I see it—what I'd hoped wouldn't be there, what I'd hoped I had imagined—the wreckage and the short trail of tire marks leading up to it.

Fifteen gallons of gasoline is spewing from my 4Runner's ripped fuel line—a deluge running down the bridge. The other car is most frightening—a pluming inferno mere feet from the stream of gas. All at once, I am in a haze, trying to remember how I got here.

After filling my car with gas just off Highway 4 in Martinez, I drove up Cummings Skyway, jerking my head for glimpses of the water and the bridge in the distance. I was messing with the radio, trying to find a good song on one of my favorite stations. Frustrated with the selection, I pulled out my phone to connect it to the auxiliary cord attached to the stereo. I was distracted with one hand on the wheel and one hand on my phone, reaching for the cord. It was dangerous, but I was invincible, or maybe just invulnerable—oblivious to the fragility of my mortality.

Finally I connected the auxiliary cord and, with one tap of my phone, the perfect song, "Undiscovered" by James Morrison, hummed through the speakers. It felt inspirational, as if I was in a movie montage synced to my favorite playlist. I was driving, or what felt like floating, across the Carquinez Strait, through Vallejo, and up to Highway 37 with what seemed like a fun evening ahead. A fun evening was not ahead. But the Napa River Bridge was.

The incline of the bridge created a dangerous illusion, leaving a blind spot a few car lengths in front of me. It was, on this day, more dangerous than trying to connect my phone to an auxiliary cord while driving.

I drove up the arching bridge, expecting to make it to the other side like any other driver, but at the top—a spot of which I hadn't seen—a car had stopped in my lane. Never in my life has so much happened in so few seconds. There was the throttle, the brake, the crash, the flames, the explosion, then, the sizzling sound. It's a familiar sound—you could spend your entire life hearing it—an overcooked piece of meat in the oven, a flaming marshmallow in a campfire—but once you associate it with burning human flesh, it changes you.

* * *

I gape at the flaming car, its small frame engulfed by a giant, billowing cloud of thick, black smoke. Every few seconds a strong breeze whips up and blows away a patch of smoke, revealing the charred, almost molten metallic exterior of the car, and the interior—a dark, shadowy tomb of helplessness and death.

I'm in shock, utterly paralyzed, afraid to move, scared that anything I do will cause further damage, that if I take another step, or so much as breathe the wrong way, I will end someone else's life.

A middle-aged man runs up to me on the bridge. He's out of breath and looks as disturbed as I feel.

"Someone's trapped in there." He points to the burning car, then frantically looks over at my 4Runner. The driver's door is wide open, and the front end looks like a folded up accordion. "Where's the other driver?"

"I am the other driver." My voice is hoarse, like I've been yelling, but I haven't said a word until now.

"That's your car?" the man asks, gesturing to my totaled 4Runner. I nod, and he looks at me worriedly. "Are you okay?"

"I think so."

"You're not okay. Look at your car," he says. "You should sit down. An ambulance will be here soon."

In search of comfort, I retreat to my spot on the bridge railing. But there's no comfort there, nor anywhere. Not even the vast, calm marsh in the background can soothe the turbulence of this moment. I feel empty, like I've lost something. Something priceless. What innocence I had is gone now that I've seen the destruction that can happen to a person, how a body and the life it holds can be destroyed so quickly and so violently.

On the road behind me, cars have stopped—drivers and passengers watching in awe, some holding up their phones, taking pictures of the giant fireball beside me. I want them to go away, or better, I want to go back in time, rewind to an hour ago and just stay there. Then I wouldn't have to think about all the things that could have diverted my fate away from this moment—a phone call, a stoplight, a bathroom break, and the one failed diversion that haunts me most: a soy corn dog.

Before I left, I had passed on an offer from David, my friend Ian's dad, to enjoy the meatless snack.

"Hey, how 'bout a corn dog before you go?" he'd asked. "They're almost ready . . ."

"No, thanks. I gotta get going. I have tickets to the Giants game and need to stop at home first."

"Okay, maybe next time," David had replied.

I smiled and nodded, then asked, "Why do you eat soy corn dogs instead of the real ones?"

"I like them," he said.

I should've stayed; I like them, too. It wasn't twenty-four hours earlier that David and I had shared an almost identical conversation, except then I had stopped to relax and eat. It was a small yet fateful part of an enjoyable weekend reconnecting with friends, but now it seems so long ago, like a story from a bygone era.

* * *

Under the railing there's a small gap of air before the bridge turns to concrete. Wispy clouds float above, shading me from the sun while I crouch down and rest my forehead on the cold metal railing, my chin on the grainy concrete. It's the closest thing to a hiding spot that I can find, a slice of shelter away from the thumbtacks and the mayhem surrounding me. I dig my phone out of my jeans and call my mom. She doesn't answer. I keep calling, then remember that she's off on a camping trip away from cell phone service. I try my dad. He won't be here for several hours. I call David and Ian. They'll meet me at the hospital.

I put my phone away and look up to see an ambulance and a fire truck zig-zagging through traffic on the bridge. Once they arrive, the firefighters get to work putting out the flames on the other car. Some of them appear detached, apathetic even, and without a trace of compassion, while others seem sympathetic but are more puzzled than worried. The Highway Patrol officers are also on the scene and, after a lead from a witness, home in on me with both fervor and confusion. One of them tests my motor skills to see if I'm drunk in the middle of the day. Hard to blame him; it's his job. Finally he clears me to leave and I get into the ambulance.

On the ride to the hospital, the paramedic is sincere but not as comforting as a friend. We arrive at the hospital—Solano something. Remembering the name of a hospital is like trying to remember the name of a street in the desert—they all look the same, and you're too focused on getting the hell out of there to care.

After stepping out of the ambulance, I walk into the emergency room without help, looking healthier than the nurse waiting to put me on a gurney. Once I'm settled, an ER doctor takes a seat next to me. He's a confident man, probably in his early-forties, with gray hair and dark bags under his eyes.

"Jameson, like the whiskey?" the doctor asks, looking at my name on a form.

"No," I say. "My name is spelled with an *i*, not an *e*."

"Looks like they got it wrong on your form. It happens a lot. I'll fix it for you in a bit." He smiles at me. "We have some juice and crackers coming for you. That's all there is at the moment."

"Thanks," I say.

"So, Jamison, you have an abrasion on your forehead . . . how do you feel? Any dizziness? Or pain in the rest of your body?" the doctor asks.

"No, I'm fine," I say. The truth is that I don't know if I'm fine. I'm still in shock, too jacked up on adrenaline to know whether I'm okay. There could be a gaping wound in my head and I probably wouldn't feel it.

"Well, you can thank your airbag for that," the doctor says.

"I didn't have one."

The doctor looks surprised. "Oh, well, that's miraculous for such a serious accident." He glances down at his clipboard. "Okay, so we're going to keep you for a couple hours just to make sure you don't have anything serious going on. Now, I know it may not be the same, but I have some idea of what you're going through. I was in a pretty bad car accident myself—I woke up in the hospital with a broken jaw, concussion, and a bunch of shattered bones."

"Oh," I mumble, staring off in the distance. I wish I had woken up in the hospital instead of witnessing the horrors of this car accident.

"Who knows why people like you and me are spared. It could be to finish what we started in life, or it could just be plain luck. I'll bet you don't have the slightest idea why this happened, or maybe it doesn't matter to you, but I bet at least part of you is wondering why you're still alive—remarkably so—and why the other guy isn't. It's all yours to sort out … or not, your choice," the doctor continues, leaning forward in his chair and resting his elbows on the gurney. "But, Jamison, if you're anything like me, there's a good chance you're going to get so frustrated trying to make sense of all the bad things that happen in your life, especially this, that you may want to give up. Maybe you already do, but if you're as smart as you seem, in that moment everything will make as much sense as it needs to."

The doctor rubs his face, a red gloss coating his tired, sincere eyes. Talking to him makes me realize something: crashing into that car on the bridge was incredibly unlucky, but of all the people fate brings to this hospital, I am one of the lucky ones. I get to go home. My life will go on.

The doctor pats my leg, gets up, and walks away. He comes back a few minutes later, delicately places his hand on my wrist, and attaches a laminated hospital bracelet—which, thanks to him, has the correct spelling of my name. "I got you taken care of," he says.

It's a small but meaningful gesture—knowing that this doctor has an idea of what I'm going through, and cares enough to spell my name right, brings me some peace. He may not be able to take away my pain, but he doesn't have to, having someone here who empathizes with me is enough.

CHAPTER 2

———

My Way of Coping

July 14, 2009

The pain in my head and chest kicked in about twelve hours after I was released from the hospital. I didn't expect to be in that much pain, but it made sense that I was. I did, after all, crash head-on into another car on the highway.

Even so, the ER doctor didn't do any major tests—no MRI or even bloodwork. Not that I wanted to do tests. I wanted to go home and avoid the nurses and doctors poking and prodding at me. I would've stayed if they had insisted, but they didn't. Probably because my only noticeable injuries were a small abrasion on my head from slamming into the steering wheel and a contusion on my chest from the seatbelt, both of which felt like someone had beaten me with a baseball bat the next day. But now, a month later, I feel fine. So fine, in fact, that I'm going to the gym at one thirty in the morning.

Leaving my house now will get me to the gym by two and done with my workout before the sun comes up. After taking a pre-workout supplement, a proprietary blend of unregulated amphetamine-like substances, I grab my water jug and gym bag and walk out to the car, a Ford Explorer that I've borrowed from a friend.

An eerie silence blankets the car as I sit in the driver's seat, anxiously gripping the steering wheel, rubbing my fingers on its plastic surface. I take a long breath and jam the keys in the ignition, then close my eyes and quickly twist my wrist. The engine revs, and my body stiffens. The thumping in my chest and the sweat on my hands tells me that this isn't going to be easy. My face feels hot, and my breathing is rapid and heavy. I try to catch my breath, but there isn't enough oxygen in the world to soothe my labored lungs.

I turn the car off, pull the keys from the ignition, and look at my phone. It doesn't matter what time it is or whether there are any notifications, I just need a distraction—somewhere for my mind to go until I can compose myself. I lean forward and rest my forehead on the steering wheel. There's a gap between the top and the middle of the wheel. It's smaller than the gap under the railing on the Napa River Bridge, but it serves a similar purpose—a place to hide from the chaos in my life. I so desperately want to crawl into that little space and stay there until this moment passes, until I'm no longer afraid to drive.

Eventually I push my fear aside long enough to drive toward the gym. But I still feel uneasy. It's the first time I've driven alone in a car since the accident, and watching bad drivers on the road makes the feeling worse. The car in front of me keeps swerving, almost rhythmically, as if the driver is partially in control and coherent but distracted, maybe trying to connect an auxiliary cord or something dumb like that. I can't take my eyes off the car and its reckless swaying.

Look at this idiot. He's going to lose control, bounce off the median, and smash through the windshield, taking out five other cars and killing everyone in a bloody, broken-glass-everywhere, fiery wreck.

I've been imagining car crashes a lot lately. I don't actually see them; they're more like quick, nightmarish flashes in my mind's eye, usually stirred by the antagonistic voice in my head. Last week on the Richmond Bridge, I imagined the car I was in had careened over the railing and into the water. Right as I was taking a last gulp of air, trapped in the corner of the capsized car, my inner voice brought me back to a reality of taillights on the bridge.

The voice is very much my own, but it's more abrasive than any side of my personality that I outwardly show. I won't pretend to know what it means—maybe it's a result of feeling helpless in a situation that I can't control, maybe it's the voice of the older brother that I never had, maybe it's underlying guilt for having killed someone in the car accident, or maybe I just don't want to know what it is.

Come on, don't get all analytical about it. Everyone has a voice in their head. Besides, this is nothing new. I've always been here knocking around your mind.

I'll admit, I'm a little messed up right now. Okay, I'm really messed up right now. I can't even look at a car without feeling anxious, and I've cried more in the past few days than I have in the past few years. The therapist I've been seeing says that's normal; it's all part of the coping process. That's about the only helpful thing he's said though. Usually he just talks about sports, which I wouldn't mind, except I'm paying him one hundred dollars an hour.

Besides, I've found a more cost-effective way of working through my trauma. Lately I've been going to the gym in the middle of the night because every emotion that I have right now must be filtered through the endorphin-tinted lens of exercise.

There's nobody at the front desk when I walk in the gym, so I pull out my wallet and mockingly flash my membership card to the obnoxiously happy cardboard employee. I return the card to its place in my wallet, next to the laminated hospital bracelet, which I wore for a week after the car accident, then folded up in my wallet for safe keeping.

After passing the front desk, I routinely whisk my way through the gym. It's empty and illuminated, humming with electricity from the sea of exercise equipment, just as it will be when the early birds arrive in a few hours. There are many things to love about an empty gym. There is peace, comfort, and an almost indescribable sense of privilege just to be there, like standing in an empty stadium, or witnessing the calm of the ocean after a storm. For me, it conjures up a rare, personal, and oddly emotive feeling, like finding comfort watching a single light in a dark landscape.

The gym is where I'm supposed to be, where my energy belongs. It's my cathedral, the sacred place I find my purpose and properly worship the things I care about most in this world—fitness and bodybuilding. It's where my coping, my healing, and all my other inner processes are meant to happen, and for good reason.

With no one else around, I feel free to fully be myself. There are no sweaty alpha males sizing me up in the mirrors, tacitly challenging my masculinity with their condescending looks. There's nobody asking me about the best protein powder to buy, or how much creatine to take. This is my chance to let go of my inhibitions and be myself without having to interact with anyone.

A twenty-four hour gym is almost never empty. Even at this hour, there is usually some rebellious teen taking selfies on a recumbent bike, or an old guy air drumming on a treadmill.

Believe it or not, these are my people. They never bother me and are exceptionally comforting to share a space with.

That's because they barely exist to you. They are less than strangers; they are inanimate, like a bookshelf. You just want them to stay out of your way. It makes sense—then they can't hurt you. They won't, by some freak twist of fate, almost end you.

In the locker room, I change into an old sleeveless T-shirt and scroll through the music on my phone. The clock on the screen reads two thirty. After taking a swig of water, I untangle my earbuds while a mellow Jack Johnson song fades in, though the soothing music does little to calm my tense nerves. When I get to the weight room, I instinctively charge the dumbbell rack as if it just threw a drink in my face or insulted my family.

Or stopped its car in the middle of the highway and just sat there until you crashed into it?

Beginning with two sixty-pound dumbbells, I do chest presses, then repeat with eighties, ninety-fives, hundreds, finally finishing the last set with one hundred and ten pounds in each hand. Next is a circuit of dumbbell flies, plyometric push-ups, and cable presses. Then I do inverted push-ups with my feet against a wall. I do them mostly just to show off, even though there's no one in the gym to impress. I don't care though, I'm having fun—this is my playground, and I have it all to myself.

The last exercise of the workout, weighted push-ups, is my favorite. It starts with two forty-five-pound plates on my back. Getting them into place without a spotter is difficult. I shimmy and wiggle both plates behind my back until I feel stable enough to start doing the push-ups. After ten reps, I fall to the floor. The polished concrete is sticky and covered in debris, but getting up right now isn't an option. Removing the plates from my back would be pointless, so they stay put until the next set while I stare at the dirty floor in front of my face.

It may seem like a miserable situation, but I love it. It's almost five in the morning, and I'm sprawled out with ninety pounds pinning me to the floor, my mouth about an inch from a dried up collection of other people's sweat.

There's no place I'd rather be.

CHAPTER 3

Still Healthy

August 29, 2009

The bathtub is sprinkled with what looks like little mounds of dirt but are actually clumps of hair—some red, some blond, others black and brown. I'm shaving my body hair, all of it, for a fitness modeling photo shoot later today. Shaving my back and butt is the hardest part, and it's usually impossible without help from a friend. This is one of those situations when having more flexibility would be useful, especially since there is no worse question to ask a friend than, "Will you shave my ass?" Luckily my friends are open-minded.

When I'm done, I wash the mounds of hair down the drain, then get dressed and eat some lunch before I borrow a friend's car and drive down to San Francisco for the photo shoot. The drive is longer than I feel comfortable doing by myself—I'm nervous the entire hour that I'm on the road as I imagine crashing into the cars in front of me, violent explosions rocking me to my core. But I press on because I'm determined not to let the trauma from the car accident dictate how I live my life.

I arrive in San Francisco and meet the photographer at Crissy Field, then hide behind his car and change into a pair of tiny spandex shorts with sweatpants over them. Today I will mostly be doing fitness modeling, though recently I've also been doing some lifestyle and underwear work. I have yet to make any money at it, but in building my portfolio, I'm hoping to be featured on a major magazine cover like *Muscle & Fitness*, and at some point in the future, I want to be a fitness personality with my own TV show.

Despite my fake tan, carefully applied makeup, and smooth skin, I aim to blend in with the other people enjoying their Saturday outings in San Francisco. The only problem is that I don't blend in. There are two noticeable types of people at Crissy Field today—locals and tourists—and a half-naked fitness model fits into neither category.

I ditch my flip-flops and sweatpants, then discreetly duck between two industrial storage containers and strike a pose. The photographer gives me instructions and clicks his camera as I transform myself into a fabricated version of masculinity.

Then I hear footsteps around the corner. The photographer tosses me my sweatpants and we try to act natural—just two guys inspecting the structural elements of the storage containers, one with a camera, the other without a shirt on.

A family of four walks by without a second glance at the oddity of the situation. They must be immune to such things. Between the Pride Parade, Bay to Breakers, and all the other wild events in the city, our guerrilla photo shoot probably looks quite tame to passersby. If I get a dirty look today, there is a decent chance it'll be because I'm not entirely naked.

We arrive at the last location, Twin Peaks. I walk to the top of a steep hill and look down at the crowded city below, catching breathtaking views in every direction—rows of tall buildings and the deep blue water surrounding them. Looking out over the city gives me the unusual feeling of standing on top of the world while only being a small part of it. I don't know whether I'm more intimidated or more inspired, but at least I'm in a beautiful city, doing something I enjoy, and even if I feel small in this moment, I'm still healthy, still finding my way in the big world sprawled out before me.

CHAPTER 4

Just a Façade

September 19, 2009

As I walk to the gym, the Sonoma County air is refreshing—wet and dewy with a light breeze that soothes my dry skin like a fan blowing cool mist. The hazy sunlight illuminating the moist air invigorates me, even amid the strong smell of manure from the surrounding dairy farms. It's a pungent, earthy smell that assaults my nostrils, though after two years of living with it, I've almost gotten used to it. So much so, my friends and I jokingly call it the "Sonoma Aroma."

Once I arrive at the gym, I complete one of my usual three-hour workouts, then wait outside for my roommate, James, to pick me up. James has been my friend since middle school. He's kind and generous, and since my 4Runner was totaled in the accident, he has let me borrow his car several times and given me countless rides, usually back to Martinez, where we both grew up. On these trips, he's been consider-ate enough, without even being asked, to avoid driving over the Napa River Bridge. I haven't been back to the bridge since the accident, mostly because I'm afraid that returning to the scene will trigger even more anxiety and flashbacks than I'm already experiencing. I'm just not ready to voluntarily relive the trauma. I am, however, ready to replace my totaled car.

James drops me off at the bank, where the owner of my soon-to-be Nissan Xterra is waiting. I withdraw seven thousand dollars—the entirety of my financial aid disbursement for the semester, which means that, for the next several months, I'll be living solely on my part-time income as a fitness instructor.

The owner of the Xterra accepts my money, neatly packed into a bulging envelope, then she signs the pink slip, hands over the keys and, just like that, the car is mine. Holding the metal keys in my hand is exhilarating, and I feel relieved to no longer have to ask friends for rides. But the feeling is a bit more complicated, a little terrifying, actually. Now that I have a car again, I can no longer rely on the excuse of not having one. If I'm feeling anxious, I can still ask my friends for rides, but I'll have to admit to them—and to myself—that I'm too rattled to drive on my own. And I'm just too proud to do that.

But maybe it won't be an issue. Sometimes driving doesn't bother me. If there's no traffic, and I'm just cruising on an open road, I can relax without feeling traumatized by the car accident. But other times, when I have no choice but to go through heavy traffic on a busy road, driving can feel like torture, stuck in my own reoccurring nightmare.

Luckily, my inaugural drive of the Xterra is on relatively empty roads. I ride through Rohnert Park, where I live and go to school at Sonoma State University. It's a small city about an hour's drive north of San Francisco. When I tell people where I live, I usually just say, "Sonoma," since Rohnert Park is in Sonoma County and most people know the broader area as part of wine country. It's easier to explain than saying that I live in a small city most people have never heard of.

Rohnert Park is a very structured place, with many of the local laws and regulations conforming to strict social norms. Once I went around hanging up flyers for the group fitness classes that I teach, and then I later found them all taken down by an aggressive neighborhood watch member. Even the names of the neighborhoods adhere to a strict code—each section of the city is named with a letter and each street within the section starts with that same letter.

On my way home, I drive through C section and several other letters of the alphabet before passing the Sonoma State campus and finally arriving at M section. From Middlebrook, I turn onto Maureen, and then drive down my street, Mary Place, a short cul-de-sac that is the epitome of suburbia. Everything on the street is insipid—driveways, houses, sidewalks, fire hydrants, lawns—it's all one big blob of vanilla ice cream.

I park the Xterra in my driveway toward the end of Mary Place and stare listlessly at the steering wheel, silently hoping that something bad doesn't happen. The onslaught of legal issues that I've been fending off could fall upon me at any moment, beginning with phone calls from the Department of Motor Vehicles, my lawyer, or the District Attorney's office. The older, highly intelligent people on these calls are so intimidating and so aggressive, they make me want to crawl into a ball and not talk to anyone. With one stroke of a pen, the District Attorney could charge me with vehicular manslaughter. I'd lose everything, be forced to drop out of school and spend tens of thousands of dollars that I don't have on additional legal fees while hoping that I would be found not guilty. Only then could I start to rebuild my life.

As a preemptive measure, so I can avoid thinking about any of this, I turn my phone off. Then I take out my wallet and find the laminated hospital bracelet. I hold it in my hand for a few seconds, rubbing its plastic seal, a sense of calm slowly washing over me. There's something comforting, however inexplicably, about the hospital bracelet. Like a battle wound, it proves that I've survived, that I'm still alive, still breathing, and nothing else really matters—certainly not all the bureaucratic bullshit that's been stressing me out. Keeping the bracelet in my new car feels like the right thing to do, instead of throwing it away or putting it in a box for a decade or two until I'm ready to get rid of everything that reminds me of the day I killed someone.

I reach up and attach the laminated bracelet to the overhead visor, just below the mirror cutout. Then I flip the visor back up and walk into the house. James has beaten me home and is sitting on the couch playing video games. I join him for a couple hours, then leave for work. This evening, I'm teaching a boot camp class that runs every Tuesday and Thursday evening at Saint Rose Catholic School in Santa Rosa, about a twenty-minute drive from my house.

About fifteen clients have signed up for the class. Most are middle-aged soccer moms who rarely show up despite having paid a monthly fee. Assuming my role as a tough trainer, however unnatural to me, I regularly message them on Facebook if they don't show up to class. When I'm in a good mood, it's usually something to the effect of: "Hey, we missed you at boot camp today. It was a great workout. Hope to see you next time!" When I'm in a bad mood, it usually goes something like: "Why weren't you at boot camp today? Everyone else was there. You paid for the classes, you should use them. Be there next time!"

With a whiteboard and equipment bag in hand, I speed walk to the blacktop to find that a few of the clients already have their shtick ready. As if I'm a comedian taking the stage, they start heckling as soon as I show up. And it seems they've been practicing.

"How come you never do the exercises with us?" a client asks. "Are you one of those 'do as I say, not as I do' trainers?"

"Do I look like one of those trainers?" I scribble the exercises on the whiteboard and hook up a pair of portable speakers to drown her out with some Black Eyed Peas.

"I guess not, but you do look cocky," the woman says over the music, and the other clients start cackling.

"Oh, okay. Remind me to take away your discount next class," I quip, looking at her deadpan. "If I do the exercises with you, then I can't point out all the mistakes you're making, like how your torso leans too far forward on squats, or how your knee goes past your toes on lunges. These are all things that can cause injuries."

"Yeah, yeah, but can we get back to how narcissistic you are?" the woman says with a grin on her face.

"You're relentless." I shake my head and try to ignore her.

What did you expect? You haven't told her, or anyone besides your family and close friends, about the car accident. You can't expect people to be gentle with you all the time, especially if you don't tell them what's going on. They look at you and see a healthy fitness trainer unfazed by everything. They don't know that you're struggling and doing all you can to make it seem like you're okay. They don't know that it's all a façade.

CHAPTER 5

Venting of Internal Monologue

March 4, 2010

Tonight I'm in a support group as part of my psychology class at Sonoma State, and it's my turn to share a traumatic experience. I'm hoping it will be more therapeutic than the one-on-one sessions that I've done with the therapist who likes to talk about sports a little too much.

I've agreed to discuss the car accident with the seven other people in the group on one condition: I will not stand in front of them and spill a sad sob story all over the linoleum floor. There will be no crying, no feeling sorry for myself, no blabbering on about my suffering. I will be pragmatic in talking about the car crashes I imagine while driving, and the excessive hours that I spend in the gym trying to numb the emotional pain I feel from the accident.

People in the group will probably ask questions, and I'll try to be transparent with my answers, because all I really want is to confide my thoughts to someone who understands what I'm going through, someone who isn't getting paid to care about my problems. I'll tell the group about how surreal life was that first night after coming home from the hospital—how I sat around with friends, watching a sketch comedy show on TV, and how it all felt so normal, but uncomfortably so—everyone was calm and relaxed while I was a smoldering ball of emotion. *Why weren't they yelling and blasting heavy metal music and doing lines of cocaine and punching each other?*

I will use my time in front of the group to talk about how I froze up in my DMV hearing, how I just sat in the dingy government office quietly reliving the accident in my mind, and how I could've had my license taken away if my mom hadn't hired a lawyer to speak on my behalf.

In front of this group of my peers, I will finally open up and talk about the things that I've been holding back, the things that I purposely haven't told anyone. I'm ready to purge, ready to unload the thoughts that have been haunting me. This is, after all, what these groups are for—the airing of dirty laundry, the uninhibited venting of internal monologue and, of course, the desperate search for validation. At least that's why I'm here tonight. I'm here for every second of this hand-holding, soul-searching group therapy session because I want—maybe even need—to do it for myself.

But I refuse to lose my composure and become emotional, like the guy speaking before me. He's a large man, probably in his mid twenties, with a thin and patchy brown beard. The more he talks about his trauma, the more uncomfortable it gets—uncomfortable for him, uncomfortable for the group, uncomfortable for the inanimate objects in the room. His story is wavering and vague, something about his childhood, something to do with his parents, his dad. He pauses and tries to talk more, but only tears come out, lots of sniffly man tears, then more ambivalence.

My goal for the next half hour is to not become that guy. I will stand up confidently, with my stack of notes, and speak candidly. I will mention the physical pain of being in a serious car accident—the chest contusion and throbbing I felt in my head the next day—as well as the mental anguish of not remembering what I had been doing in the moments before the crash. Had I driven over the sixty-five miles-per-hour speed limit? Had I looked in the rearview mirror before I crashed? Was that why I didn't see the car stopped in front of me? I will try to answer these questions and talk about how the small discrepancy between the speed limit and how much faster I thought I was going put me at fault on the official accident report.

The truth is you don't know how fast you were driving, but stupidly, you put yourself at fault by saying you were going seventy miles per hour. You're lucky the District Attorney was busy with capital crimes; you could have gone to prison.

I will also discuss how sickening it is to attach monetary value to a life, how the deceased's family deserved much more than the thirty thousand dollars my insurance paid out, and how if I had just bought a better policy, they would have received more money, or so the claims adjuster had said. I may tell the group how that same claims adjuster hired an investigator who checked my phone records and found that I wasn't texting or talking on my phone while I was driving, and contrary to the Highway Patrol's report, he deemed me not to be at fault.

Then I will talk about the emotional grenades that keep detonating in my life, how sometimes I can't drive in a car because it makes me too anxious, and how I have to look away or walk out of the room whenever I see an accident on TV and in movies. I will mention that I often vex myself by calling it "my accident," when I wish so vehemently to relinquish all ownership of it.

I'll also speak about the remorse I feel for the man I killed, how I knew nothing about him until I read the accident report, and how I've since forgotten his name and everything else I read about him.

Maybe you don't want to know anything about him.

As I finish speaking, I will be insightful, introspective, but not prolix, and the people in the group will respond with lots of hugs and handshakes. I will feel better, relieved to have purged myself of all the emotions I've been harboring. Then I will move on with my life—my new car, my job, my final year of college and, of course, my fitness and bodybuilding aspirations.

CHAPTER 6

My Totem

May 8, 2010

For the last several months, I've been preparing for a natural bodybuilding competition, and today I get to see if all my hard work will pay off. My ass is shaved, my food is prepped, my self-tanner applied, and my posing trunks—a step up or down from a thong, depending on your view—are hidden under my sweatpants. And these are just the preparations I've made today. I've spent the last several weeks working out as much as possible, restricting my caloric intake, and tapering my fluid consumption to thirty-two ounces a day with the purpose of dehydrating my muscles so they're more visible when I'm posing on stage.

Keith and Tony, two of my friends from the gym, are carpooling with me to the competition. Keith, a bulky, clean-cut man in his late-twenties with a shaved head and wiry glasses, has decided not to compete. But Tony, a tall, muscular redhead also in his late-twenties, has transformed himself from pale and freckled to bronzed effigy with a few coats of self-tanner. I have essentially done the same, except I look more like an Oompa Loompa with raccoon eyes.

We hit the road, cruising through Rohnert Park, the happiest bodybuilders in the world. We pass S section, C section, D section, and finally make it to the commercial part of town near Highway 101. Tony is giving Keith shit about not competing, and as entertaining as their conversation is, all I'm thinking about is the big, greasy pizza I get to eat at the end of the day, my just reward for starving my body over the past several weeks.

We're stopped at the last intersection before the highway, when A cool breeze blows through my fingers tapping on the car door as the morning sun peeks through the groves of redwood trees lining the busy road. The light is warm on my face, stinging my tired eyes, so I flip down the overhead visor to shield them from the sun. On the visor, attached by a paper clip, is my laminated hospital bracelet.

I glance over at the rearview mirror and see a large vehicle rushing past traffic. It's really moving. It looks like an ambulance trying to get through the gridlock. I turn my head to get a better look. It's not an ambulance but a truck that has hopped the curb and is now speeding across the sidewalk beside us. Pedestrians are running, jumping out of the way of the massive vehicle barreling down on them. *Bam!* The truck takes out a road sign, sending a jarring sound ringing through the air. Then it takes out a streetlamp and another road sign, launching debris in every direction.

This is the worst timing, the worst possible timing, to imagine a car crash. I'm trying, really trying, to keep it together, but it feels like my grip on reality is slipping, falling further away with each passing second.

What do you want? A trophy? Someone to give you an award for trying to keep it together? You have to stop imagining these car crashes. They're not healthy or constructive. You are only making things harder for yourself by letting the car accident interfere with your life.

I shake my head and bang my hands on the steering wheel. Then I look outside and see the truck still there, whizzing through the intersection, narrowly missing cars, people, traffic lights. I'm still here, I think, holding my breath and clawing the steering wheel, on the verge of flinging myself out of the car and running down the street, frantic, like a dehydrated meth addict in the middle of summer.

The truck hops another curb and flies straight into an embankment.

Okay, you obviously can't control yourself right now. You should have Keith or Tony drive the rest of the way. Either that or, right here and now, realize that the accident on the bridge is never going to happen to you again, except by reliving it through these episodes. The guy you killed was either really unlucky, or he wanted to die. What are the odds his car stalled out in the one place on the bridge that you couldn't see up ahead? And he didn't get out of his car, put the hazard lights on, or even try to pull over to the shoulder. He just fucking sat there. He wasn't trying to kill himself, he was waiting for you to do it for him. You will never see that on an official report, but it's the best explanation you are going to get, and because it's your own, it is the only one that truly matters. Now get over it or give over the keys.

I pull over to the side of the road. My hands are shaking, and my heart is beating so fast it feels like my chest is about to cave in. Tears brim from my eyes as I shut the engine off and yank the keys from the ignition. I consider who to hand them to, Keith or Tony, and how to explain that I'm too shaken up, too emotionally damaged to keep driving. Surely they will question why I've delayed our trip, why I'm crying, and what the hell is wrong with me. But I don't know if I'm ready to describe my tragic past, to answer questions about what a burning body looks like and if an exploding car really does what it does in the movies. Still, I will try to convey my reality to Keith and Tony and convince myself that I don't want their sympathy or attention, except why else would I be making such a big deal about my trauma? At last, I prepare myself for the big reveal, the stupid mood-spoiling, day-ruining, all-about-me big reveal. I take a long breath and turn to my friends. But they're gone.

Keith and Tony have disappeared, their seats empty, car doors swung wide open. Through the windshield, I see the truck; it's still there, crashed against the embankment. Then the driver's door springs open, and a dog comes vaulting out. Finally I see Keith and Tony running toward the truck, futilely trying to corral the dog as a large man plops to the ground. He's lying on his back with his knees in the air, holding his chest, appearing to be having a heart attack. He takes out his cell phone, likely to call 9-1-1, but he abruptly hangs up as if the exertion of holding the phone to his ear is too much, or maybe he just realized that fifty people already called when he ran over the first street sign.

Still in the driver's seat, I frantically feel along the center console, the dashboard, the door, searching for a totem—something to show me that this is actually happening. I need to prove to myself that this is real and not some elaborate, far-from-funny prank my subconscious is playing on me.

I look up. The overhead visor is still flipped down, and there it is—my totem, my own personal reality check right in front of me. I unpin the thin plastic hospital bracelet and feel the air bubbles in the lamination, the dulled adhesive on the corners. I read the faded letters of my name. Like the person it identifies, the bracelet is worn and tattered but somehow still intact.

CHAPTER 7

Emotional Gunk

September 10, 2010

It's been several months since I watched the truck drive off the road on my way to the bodybuilding competition, and I'm still haunted by it. And the rest of the day didn't go much better. I tried to shake it off, but when I got to the competition, it became clear that I was unfocused and overmatched by older, seasoned bodybuilders, like Tony, who walked away with every possible award that night, as if the trophy store went out of business and gave him its entire inventory.

Then, after we went out for pizza and way too much beer, I woke up the next morning with a hairless body, a fake tan, and the worst hangover of my life. I was planning on doing another competition later this year, but my body is too run down, too tired and sluggish. So I've decided to take a break from the competitions. I'm still going to work out like I always do, but I'm also going to try to let loose and have more fun.

Tonight James and I are playing a drinking game with our roommate, Thomas, a muscular ultimate frisbee player with short brown hair and freckles scattered over his pale skin like little flecks of gold. Since Thomas moved in with us this summer, he has quickly become one of my best friends. Once a week, we drive up to Trader Joe's in Santa Rosa to go grocery shopping together. Last time, we bought pizza dough and made a deep dish, splitting it in half with his side full of pepperoni and my side filled with kale.

When we're not cooking pizzas, we usually play video games or watch documentaries. We often talk about making a documentary of our own once we graduate, even though we know nothing about filmmaking. The closest we've come to filming a documentary was when we made a YouTube video called "Battle of the Blender," in which we pranked each other by putting unusual items in our communal blender as the other person was making a protein shake. The video ended with Thomas trying to put a barstool in my shake, proving that he has a unique sense of humor that makes it effortless for us to be friends.

After I've had a couple of beers with Thomas and James, another one of my friends, Kendra, arrives with a much needed thirty-pack of the cheapest beer a college student could dream of. Kendra is the definition of an old soul, and her personality is as vivacious as the curls in her brown hair. She's the type of person I could get along with in pretty much any situation—a four-hour class, a raging party, a trip to the grocery store, even a preschool with frantic children running around, screaming and stomping on my feet.

Kendra and Thomas, and James and I have paired off to play a partner drinking game called corners. The four of us each stand next to a corner of a long plywood table in the garage. In front of each of us is a pyramid of three cups filled with beer. In the middle of the table is a lone cup with water in it. The game is rapid fire, shooting a ping-pong ball diagonally across the table into our partner's cups.

The game starts with James making a cup. I pass it to Kendra to drink, and she gives me a begrudging look. I shoot, make a cup, and James passes it to Thomas to drink. That's pretty much how the rest of the game goes until James and I have made all our cups and only need to bounce the ball in the middle cup to win. It's surprisingly difficult, considering we're not even drunk.

Thomas razzes us about being college students who can't do something a first-grader could, then Kendra makes a cup, and I drink it. Kendra and Thomas sink three more balls into the cups, which James and I quickly chug. The beer is cold, tasteless, surprisingly filling, and absolutely littered with tiny debris gathered from the ball, which makes frequent contact with the dirty garage floor. The beer keeps coming until we have only a one-cup lead, and bouncing the ball in the middle cup feels like throwing a ring off a moving carousel.

Finally, James bounces the ball in for the win, and we celebrate our victory by each taking two shots of Jameson. Kendra leaves, then Thomas, James, and I shotgun some beers, and I cap the night off with a pinch of chewing tobacco as we sit on top of the sound wall in the backyard.

Thomas sits next to me on the wall. We look out over the street behind our house and find a rare opportunity to talk about things we wouldn't bring up when we're sober, things like car accidents. Thomas tells me that he, too, was in a bad car accident and had to cope with physical and emotional trauma. His accident happened several years ago, and he still has trouble coping, but it's gotten easier over time. It's comforting to talk to someone, a friend no less, who has been through a similar experience. I can see myself, like Thomas, one day getting to a place where the trauma isn't as intense and doesn't haunt me as much as it does now. It may take time, but I know I'll get to that place.

We spend a solid hour sitting on top of the wall, talking about our respective car accidents, the night air and ripe Sonoma Aroma wafting between us. I didn't realize it until now, but I've needed this. I've needed to talk to a friend, not an apathetic therapist or even the sleepy-eyed students in the group from my psychology class. I don't know if it's just the buzz from the alcohol, but talking to Thomas feels cathartic. I may always have to live with the trauma from the car accident in some form, but in this moment I don't care. Opening up and releasing the emotional gunk inside me is what I need right now.

YEAR 1

The Illness

CHAPTER 8

The Onset

November 28, 2010

It's morning and I feel a little groggy, but I'm ready to start the day. I get out of bed and make my way to the kitchen. I bump into the refrigerator and scuttle along the wall, my depth perception thoroughly askew, until I find the laminate countertop. I pour a bowl of cereal and take it outside to eat. I down the soggy grains with two crushed caffeine pills mixed in a glass of warm water. It tastes like rubber and chalk with strong notes of poison and death, but it slowly wakes me up.

I sit on the stoop in the backyard, the sound of battered tennis balls playing in full stereo from the park across the street as I eat my breakfast and flick the sleep from my eyes. The rhythmic rallying of furry neon balls puts me in an ephemeral trance just mild enough for the caffeine buzz to bring me back to reality.

I look down at the clock on my phone. It's just after eleven.

You realize you check your phone way too often, right? Looking at the time every five seconds doesn't give you control over anything. It only proves how powerless you are.

I walk back inside, get ready for the gym, and head toward the garage where my bike is patiently waiting like a faithful Labrador wagging its tail for a walk. I hop on and ride down Mary Place as the brisk November air, finally free of the Sonoma Aroma, nips at my face. It feels good. There's a full day of accomplishment ahead, a reminder of how satisfying this busy life of mine has become.

I pedal down Middlebrook, then Bodway as the Sonoma State campus appears on the horizon. My cadence is fast and full of forceful bursts. The 1980s model Univega performs effortlessly for its age. The red light at the intersection of Bodway and East Cotati breaks my rhythm, testing the Univega's worn brake pads.

Brian, a familiar face from the gym, is also stopped at the light. He pulls his newer, more expensive bike next to mine.

"Hey, Jamison," Brian says. "Are you going to the gym?" I smile and nod. "What are you working out?"

"Legs," I say.

"Nice. Me too. You want company?"

"Yeah, sure."

"Sweet," he says, giving me a smirk. "So, speaking of legs . . . How's the modeling going?"

I give him a sideways glance and quickly think of something witty to say. "Actually, there's a photo shoot coming up that would be perfect for you. Only thing is you have to grow out all your body hair, braid it, then get naked and wear one of those constable hats."

Brian laughs and shakes his head, then the light turns green and we take off, pedaling our bikes through traffic. I'm hoping that working out with Brian will help me find the groove I've been looking for since my subpar performance at the body-building competition back in May. I've had a cold at least three times since then, and I often feel sluggish and unusually tired during my workouts. My body is probably trying to tell me something—it's worn out and needs a break from the gym, but resting goes against my grain. Even after the competition, I was back lifting weights the next day, burning off the calories from the pizza and beer I had during my post-competition binge.

For me, bodybuilding is not about competing against other people; it's about competing against myself. That may be another reason why I didn't do well in the competition. I wanted to win, sure, but I cared more about pushing my body past its ever-increasing limits than I did about achieving an award-winning physique. And the two don't always correlate: working out too much can be counterproductive to bodybuilding and good health in general. My body needs rest—days without any exercise—but that's not what I want to do. I want to work out all day, every day. I want all the exercise, all the time. Working out is my addiction, my nicotine, and I don't just want a single cigarette, or even a pack—I want to smoke the whole damn carton at once. I love working out, and nothing is going to stop me from doing what I love, which is why I'm going to the gym right now.

Sunlight peeking through redwood branches illuminates remnants of the morning mist as Brian and I ride along a campus bike path. I drift behind his bike as we emerge from the grove of trees to a stampede of bustling students. Negotiating the pace of campus pedestrians apparently involves more finesse than two bodybuilders have. We both abruptly brake to avoid tumbling into the herd, our tires skidding along the cement path. Then we carefully weave in between the walkers, runners, and even a university-issued golf cart, barely making it to the other side of the intersection.

Our destination is the Sonoma State Recreation Center, but I usually just call it the gym. The two-story building has a modern design made with a wood beam awning jutting out over the main entrance. The interior is covered in stone and polished wood surfaces. It's one of the nicest gyms I've ever used. It's also where I play three intramural sports and work as a personal trainer when I'm not teaching my boot camp class in Santa Rosa.

When I walk inside the gym, it's frigid and empty like most gyms on Sunday mornings. But this morning an eerie feeling washes over me, like lying on a cold operating table counting backward from a hundred. Despite the unusual feeling, I'm ready to work out. Three hundred milligrams of caffeine is now streaming through my blood and into my brain, priming my muscles to throw some heavy weights around.

Brian and I start the workout by warming up our muscles with some foam rolling and dynamic stretches. Then Brian approaches the squat rack. He puts a forty-five-pound plate on each side of the bar and does an easy ten reps. I follow with twelve reps, then add another plate to each side so he can readily start the next set. He struggles but finishes the lift.

"There you go, man." I use my best trainer voice, hitting a note somewhere between Jack Nicholson shouting and Richard Simmons screeching. "Nice job. Was that ten reps?"

"Yeah, barely," Brian says.

"You had good form, though. That's what matters." I start my set and complete fifteen reps without help, though I struggle a bit on the last one. Brian seems reluctant as I add more weight.

"Another forty-five?" he says, approaching the squat rack.

"You got this, man," I say. "I'll spot you, then you can drop the weight on the next set. Okay?"

"Sure," Brian says, sounding unenthusiastic. He starts his set and gets the first rep easily but begins to struggle on the second.

"Come on. One more." Again, I use my trainer voice. "I got you the whole way. Let's go, man." Brian finishes the set and lets out a big breath.

"Ah, that one almost killed me," he says. "My eyes were about to pop."

"You gotta breathe. It's all about breathing," I say. "Good job, though. You got three reps. How many do you normally get at three-fifteen?"

"I've never tried before. That was a first for me. How many can you do?" he asks.

"Hopefully I can get three, but we'll see." I'll at least get three reps. Shit, I need five just to be content.

I hoist three hundred and fifteen pounds off the squat rack, my toes at a slightly obtuse angle and knees in-line with my shoulders. Then I slowly lower my hips to a ninety-degree angle, bring them back up, and repeat the exercise four more times before I begin to slow down.

"You got this," Brian says, assuming the role of the trainer. "One more, bro." He steps behind me and wraps his arms around my waist to help me lift the weight.

"No help." I shake my head.

"Okay. Okay. It's all you," Brian says. He backs away, and I barely rack the bar in time before my legs give out. Brian gives me a thumbs up, and I stumble away from the squat rack.

"That didn't feel good," I say, moving toward the nearest chair.

"Don't sit, man. Walk it off," Brian says.

But I can't walk it off. I can't walk at all. I collapse onto the chair and blankly stare at the wall. I'm weak, my head is dizzy, and my body feels poisoned, as if I've been injected with a toxin that's quickly taking over my body. I wish I could escape to a new body, or maybe just a new time when I don't feel like puking up my breakfast. I want this feeling to stop. I want to tap out. But I can't. I don't know how.

A few minutes later, I'm still staring at the wall. It looks infinite—a featureless white abyss. My brain needs more oxygen, more blood, more everything. My vision slowly fades, and the abyss gets deeper and more pervasive, sucking me into an all-consuming vortex. The powerful maelstrom continues to drag me under as my heart beats dangerously fast. It's hard to concentrate long enough to take my pulse, but I think my heart rate is around one hundred and eighty beats per minute. It's usually about forty-five beats per minute when I'm sitting down. Maybe this is what a heart attack feels like, or maybe it's a blood clot or a hemorrhage.

Come on, this isn't a heart attack. Where's the numb arm and chest pain? This is nothing. You've been through much worse, like that time you had appendicitis and still finished the workout, went to class, then work, and did another workout the next day before finally going to see a doctor. And look, you're still alive—you're more than alive; you're thriving. This is the first decent workout you've had in months. You can't give up on this. You have to finish.

I manage to move, or rather fall, to the floor. I lie with my feet propped on the chair from which I fell. I know I look dramatic and thirsty for attention, but the attention is unwanted.

Brian finishes his set and passes the proverbial baton by lowering the weight. I prop myself up under the squat rack and notice my reflection in the wall-length mirror, which looks like I'm in a carnival fun house. Lost in the starry, infinite chasm that is my vision, I feel an invisible riptide of self-doubt threaten to pull me out to sea.

Twelve reps at two hundred and seventy-five pounds is normal for me, but I'm now struggling to get five as I do the next set, my condition worsening with each movement I make. The starry shapes and bright lights have now turned to darkness; the walls have caved in, daylight is sparse, and once again I am on the floor.

You look like one of those melodramatic meat heads grunting and theatrically falling to the floor after a workout. We get it—you work out hard and have this urge to torture yourself with exercise, but nobody really gives a shit. So let's go. Get off the floor.

Lying on the ground in a stew of pain and malaise, I'm concerned for my health. I try to face-palm the pain away, but this is a new kind of pain. It jolts me and stabs at every part of my body. It's not like the pain I usually feel during a workout—the pain I have secretly thrived on, the pain that has always kept me coming back for more.

I'm unsure about what to do next. If I stop the workout now, I would be admitting defeat, but there is no foreseeable end to this rotten feeling. If this is what taking too many caffeine pills does to me, the rest are going in the trash. This will pass. It must. It always does. I have puked, bled, even passed out while lifting weights, but I have never felt this sick.

Brian and I move on to lunges. I start by grabbing two dumbbells and lunging forward with one leg, then the other, just as I've done thousands of times before. Maybe that's why I start to feel a bit better—maybe the familiarity of it all, the comfort found in a pair of dumbbells, will bring me back to health, or maybe my body has simply run out of immune responses. It could also be the increased blood flow, or maybe it's just the caffeine leaving my system. Either way, I hope it will all be over soon.

The improvement I felt doing lunges quickly fades and returns to the awful feeling that had been surging through my body. I have intense chills, and my heart feels as if it's bouncing around in my chest, like a kid on a trampoline—that is, a trampoline fenced in with razor wire and rusty nails sticking up from the bottom.

"How are you feeling, bud?" Brian asks, a look of concern on his face. I forgot he was still standing near me. My mind is foggy and full of lapses.

"Uh, not too good, but I'm hanging in there."

The nausea that was subsiding has returned, and my circulation feels like a garden hose with a kink in it, increasing volume and pressure to force through an ample blood supply. Maybe that's why my skin has gone from hot and sweaty to cold and clammy.

"Are you down for one more lift?" Brian asks.

"Okay," I say. Now I'm the one who sounds unenthusiastic.

"Do you know how to hack squat?" he asks.

I look down at the ground, take a deep breath, and nod my head.

"Okay, you go first so I can watch. I need help with my form," Brian says.

Lifting the forty-five-pound bar off the ground is as strenuous as holding a three-hundred-pound steel beam above my head. My body has never felt this weak. Each muscle movement feels like swimming in a lake with heavy clothes on, the dead weight hanging from my limbs. Halfway through the warmup set my grip slips, and the weights drop to the floor.

"What's up, man? You all right?" Brian asks. "Want to try something else?"

"No, sorry. I'm feeling like crap. It's just not my day. I'm calling it, but let's get after it again soon."

My ego will have to deal with a premature end to the workout. I walk out of the gym and look at the time on my phone, but my vision is too blurry to read what it says. My head is full of pressure, spinning and pounding with every step I take.

The temperature outside is probably in the low-seventies, a typical Sonoma County day, but my body is freezing, shaking under four layers of clothing. And to make matters worse, I can't find my bike among the dozens of others locked to the metal racks in front of the gym. All the damn things look the same. I only see a jumbled mess of blurry handlebars, seats, and tires. I'm lost and confused, but thankfully a bit of familiarity arrives just in time.

"Hey, friend!" a voice calls out from the jumbled mess. It's Kendra, her brown eyes and each curl of her hair gradually coming into focus through my blurry vision.

"Hi." I look at her and eke out a quick smile.

"What are you doing?" She smiles back.

"Looking for my bike …"

"Oh. Where'd you put it?"

"I don't remember," I reply.

"Sure you do, silly. Isn't that it over there? The old blue one?" Kendra points to my bike locked to a metal pole a few yards away.

"Thanks," I say.

"Wanna ride with me?" Kendra asks with a smile on her face. I nod, then unlock and slowly mount the Univega.

Kendra talks casually as we ride home together. Concentrating on her words feels almost impossible, but luckily I don't need to understand them to be comforted. Giving in to the moment, to the unknown, I stop fighting my worsening symptoms and just focus on the humming coming out of her mouth. The soft vibrations of Kendra's voice brings me some peace, as much peace as there is to be found with an ailing body.

I barely make it home, then sit in a corner of my room and stare at the wall like a zombie. Some time passes—I'm not sure how long—and I forget where Kendra went or what I did with my bike.

Damn, maybe something is wrong with you. Maybe you're not just looking for attention.

More time passes and I haven't moved. I'm still sitting motionless in a corner of my room. Thomas is now standing in the doorway, but again, I'm having serious concentration problems. He's asking me a question.

"Jamison? Are you okay?"

"I . . . I don't know, it kinda feels like—"

Thomas interrupts me. "You don't look good, man. You're really pale."

"Yeah, I don't feel good." I close my eyes and try to imagine myself feeling better.

"What do you feel like?" he asks.

"What?" I open my eyes and dizzily look up at Thomas. His words sound like someone with a bad phone connection—lots of white noise with spurts of clarity.

"What do you feel?"

"Uh. My heart is beating really fast. I have chills and nausea, and I feel really dizzy. There are weird shapes, blotches everywhere, and it's hard to make out what you're saying."

"Did you take your temperature?" Thomas asks.

"I don't have a thermometer."

"Shoot, I don't have one either. Do you want me to take you to the hospital?" he asks.

"No, no, I'll be fine."

"Okay, but do you want me to get you anything? Some food or something?" Thomas asks. I think for a second, then listlessly look across the room at my backpack.

"The protein shake in my backpack might help." I point to the bag on the other side of the room.

"Sure, man. Here you go," he says, handing me the plastic bottle. "I'll check on you in a bit."

Thomas leaves my room, and I warily crawl into bed. Moving is painful. I get under the covers and try to rest, but the chills won't let up, and my accelerated heart rate makes it impossible to relax. All I can do is curl up into a ball and hope that I will feel better tomorrow.

CHAPTER 9

Urgent Care

November 29, 2010

It's a beautiful fall day. The birds are chirping, the sun is shining, but driving to urgent care feels like a slow and painful death. Yesterday morning I was healthy and feeling good, then out of nowhere I felt like I had the worst case of the flu. Last night the nausea was relentless, and the chills and pain rippling through my body kept me awake. I only got a couple hours sleep and woke up today feeling the same, if not worse.

When I get to urgent care, the waiting room is full of sick toddlers, elderly folk, and hungover twentysomethings. I tell the receptionist that I'm not feeling well, and a nurse ushers me from the waiting room. She has brown hair, a quiet voice, and looks about ten years older than me. She has me sit on a gurney behind a small curtain to give me a sense of privacy in a room full of people.

The nurse takes my vitals. "Okay, Jamison. You have a slight fever, and your heart rate is a little elevated, but nothing to worry about. Your blood pressure is normal," she says softly.

"But I don't feel normal," I say.

"Have you ever had seasonal depression or anxiety?" the nurse asks. "It could be something like that."

I give her a shrug. "I get anxious sometimes, but I've never really been depressed."

"Okay, well, I'll let you talk to the doctor about it. She will see you soon." The nurse leaves me alone behind the thin curtain.

A few minutes later, the doctor walks up and sits next to me. I tell her about my symptoms and show her the swollen lymph nodes on my neck and the strawberry-like rash on my tongue, all of which I discovered this morning. The doctor gives me a hasty physical exam, but she doesn't do blood, urine, or any other kinds of tests. She offers no definitive explanation for my condition. She does, however, reiterate the nurse's theory that I may be having depression and anxiety. The doctor says I should see my general practitioner, Dr. Gretchen, who can do a more thorough exam on me and prescribe medication, if needed.

I return home without an answer to my health problem. The whole experience at urgent care seemed pointless, like the doctor didn't want to put in the time to properly diagnose or treat me and, with a waiting room full of patients, was just trying to get me out of the way.

At home, I get a text message from Molly, my girlfriend. I met her a few months ago, and we've been spending virtually all our free time together. Her message asks if I want to go for a run, something we've been doing a lot the last several weeks. It's a way to spend time together and share our mutual love of fitness. There is nothing that I would love more than to go for a run right now, but I decline Molly's offer because I feel like I'm going to vomit and pass out every time I stand up.

An hour or so after I reply to Molly's message, I hear a knock at the door. I answer it and see Molly standing pigeon-toed on the doorstep, her dimpled face and blue eyes beaming at me as she brushes a few strands of her long blond hair out of her face.

"Hi, cutie," Molly says. She walks inside, leaving her prized Porsche parked out on the street. I wrap my arms around her, my hands gripping the back of her long-sleeved moisture-wicking shirt, which matches her black headband and spandex running pants. Hugging Molly is comforting, a nice distraction from the havoc inside my body.

"Did you go for a run?" I ask her.

"Yep. I ran home from campus, then drove here," she says. "I was going to come over first so you could run with me, but you were being a party pooper."

"Yeah, major party pooper." I smile and give Molly a kiss. Then we curl up in bed and for a long time just lie together.

Eventually Molly falls asleep, her long limbs twisted around my torso. I still feel unwell, but with her comfort, I'm finally able to relax and rest.

* * *

Waking up with Molly still nestled against me is soothing, her warm breath moistening my neck. She stirs awake and gives me a soft kiss, then we start making out and I move my hands under her shirt and along the small of her back. I kiss her neck, and she rubs her body against mine. Then she stands up and slowly slips off her shirt and pants. She does a little dance in her underwear and jumps on top of me. It turns me on, but for some reason, I can't get aroused. Nothing is happening, not the natural way it should, the way it usually does. And my symptoms are getting worse—I feel dizzy, as if I'll throw up, and my heart is racing, loudly thumping in my chest. I pretend that I'm fine, but I'm not.

Molly hovers over me, looking seductive. She takes my pants off, but I still can't get aroused. A wave of panic runs through me. It's impossible to stay calm when I'm unnerved by the thought of underperforming, or worse, not performing at all with Molly. I search for a spark—something, anything, to fulfill my sexual aspirations.

You need more than a spark; you need an antidote. Whatever this illness is, it obviously hasn't gone away. Think about it—your body was freaking out while you were doing squats yesterday. Now, less than a day later, you can't expect to have sex without a hitch. Shit, you shouldn't even try; it's a road full of embarrassment you're headed down.

Again, my heart is beating way too fast, like a cop breaking down a door, and the door is my head. I can feel fluid pumping forcefully through an artery—or maybe an organ, or something—in my abdomen. Whatever it is feels tender and swollen, as if filled with pus and covered with sores and blisters.

Stalling with the hope that a sudden rush of blood will come save the moment, I clumsily kiss Molly, pulling my pelvis away from her and pinning it awkwardly to the mattress. Molly frowns, and for a second it looks like she's going to speak, but I quickly kiss her before she says something that might add to my embarrassment. We kiss for what feels like an hour. Her soft, remarkably plump lower lip does something to me, but it's not enough to solve my problem.

We continue to make out, and I glance up at the wall above my bed where there's a poster of the Rat Pack at Carnegie Hall, each member of the group in a different posture of amusement about my erectile dysfunction. Sammy Davis, Jr. looks especially amused, and I hate him for it. On the adjacent wall, John Belushi looks dazed and confused that I can't get it up with such a gorgeous woman in my bed. The jury has spoken and I'm guilty. It feels like I've done something wrong, and now I'm shrouded in shame about my predicament. Does this happen to other guys? Guys my age? This is the first time it has ever happened to me, and yet it feels irreversible, as if now I will always, at least in my mind, have a blemish on my masculinity.

Molly reaches for me. I try to relax and give in to the moment, but the pressure from her increasingly aggressive and impatient touch leaves me squirming away.

This isn't good, man. She can't be thrilled about this. She doesn't want pillow talk—she wants passion and vigor; she wants hot, sweaty sex.

"Um, are you . . . okay?" Molly asks, as if she's been holding back, waiting for me to say something.

"Yeah," I say. "My heart is just being weird."

"What do you mean your heart is being weird?"

"It's just beating really fast. I had to stop my workout yesterday because I felt like shit. I don't know. Maybe I've been working out too much."

"You do work out a lot. You're at the gym pretty much every day. But this has never happened to us."

"I know. Something is definitely wrong," I say.

"Did you see a doctor?" Molly asks.

"I went to urgent care earlier today. It was pointless, though. The doctor just thought I was being anxious and depressed."

"Depressed? You're like the happiest person I know," Molly says.

"Yeah, I know. I think the doctor just wanted to get rid of me. I'm gonna talk to my regular doctor and see what she says. I just wish my heart would stop beating so fast. It won't slow down, even when I'm resting."

"Um, babe, that freaks me out," Molly says.

"Why?"

"Because it doesn't sound good." Molly pauses and looks down at the mattress. "I don't know about this."

"About what?" I say, my tone a little defensive.

Molly looks up at me. "About having sex. I mean, you're talking about your heart not working right, and I don't want you to, you know, die while we're doing it."

"That won't happen. It can't," I say, shaking my head. "I'm too young and healthy—guys my age don't die having sex."

Molly insists we stop, and we both get dressed in uncomfortable silence. The mood between us is awkward, but in many ways it's a relief. Had we not stopped, I might have kept trying to have sex until I actually did drop dead. I'm just not good at respecting my limits, probably because I've trained myself to always push them.

After walking Molly to the door, I watch her get into her Porsche and drive away, then I crawl back into bed and try not to think about the chaos that has become my life.

CHAPTER 10

The Only One Rattled

December 15, 2010

It's been more than two weeks since I got sick, and my health hasn't improved. Pain, weakness, and nausea are the most persistent symptoms, but the others aren't much better. My skin is clammy, and I frequently have chills. At least a couple times a day, I feel like I'm either going to puke or pass out. That's usually when I get short of breath, dizzy, disoriented, and my heart rate soars.

Dr. Gretchen, my general practitioner, a short, middle-aged woman with dark hair and remarkably straight posture, has yet to figure out why any of this has happened. I went to see her, but she didn't have a conclusive answer for my poor health, and she expressed some skepticism about my symptoms. It probably didn't help that I told her I sometimes have flashbacks and imagine car crashes while I'm driving. Now she seems to think that whatever is afflicting me is psychological, that my mind has created my illness, as if I can not only imagine car accidents but also entire illnesses. I don't think it's caused by my imagination though. I think it's caused by something pathogenic, something sophisticated and complex, something that's going to take lab tests to detect. It feels like I have a virus or bacterial illness, not something that my mind triggered.

When I mentioned this to Dr. Gretchen, she wavered a bit, but like the urgent care doctor, she still suggested that my symptoms could be caused by anxiety and depression from the car accident. I told her that I don't have depression but I do get anxiety, though working out usually makes me feel better. I also told the doctor that, in the year and a half since that fateful day on the Napa River Bridge, I've seen a therapist and participated in a support group. The trauma from the car accident is something I still struggle with, but I don't think my illness was caused by it. My current symptoms feel different than the anxiety I've experienced. I have never had a panic attack or flashback that has caused such profound weakness or made the lymph nodes on my neck tender to the touch and swollen to the size of large marbles. Anxiety has never given me a persistent fever and a strawberry-like rash covering my tongue.

I told Dr. Gretchen about these physical symptoms, but she seemed unconcerned. Her solution was to prescribe me an antidepressant medication, which she said works for anxiety too. She did do a blood draw and urine test to check for viruses, bacterial infections, and other physical illnesses, but I won't get the results for a couple weeks. I also told Dr. Gretchen that my heart rate feels especially abnormal during exercise, so she let me borrow a wearable EKG device called a Holter monitor. I'm going to use it during my next workout, in case exercise is triggering my illness.

I'm a little hesitant to wear the Holter monitor to the gym because I don't want to look weak in front of Keith and Tony and my other bodybuilding friends, but it's probably too late for that. I've already tried to work out twice this week, and each time I either had to stop prematurely or I barely finished and felt horrible afterward.

The more I try to exercise, the more obvious it is that I'm sick. The other day at the gym, I was too exhausted to lift weights, so I just sat and slowly pedaled on a recumbent bike. I tried my best to make it a good workout, but it was impossible. My body was too weak and tired. It flared up with pain, and I became dizzy and disoriented. It didn't help that when I looked over to the bike next to mine, there was an elderly man, probably a professor nearing retirement, pedaling much faster than me. He looked how I felt—frail and pale—but he was pedaling fast, smiling, and rocking out to his headphones as I struggled to pedal at all, grimacing and listening to the unsettlingly loud beat of my heart pounding through my head.

The workout lasted ten minutes, then I went home, fell asleep on the couch for three hours, woke up, ate some food, and fell back asleep until morning. I'm hoping that my workout today lasts longer; at least long enough for the Holter monitor to reveal whether something is wrong with my heart.

The Holter monitor is bulky and resembles an oversized cassette player from the 1980s. It's connected to an intricate web of wires attached to electrodes on my torso, which are not easy to hide, even under my baggiest clothes. After several minutes of trying to strap the device to my leg, I'm finally able to conceal it and look somewhat presentable. I've been reluctant to wear it because I don't want someone to see it and question me. As much as I want an answer to my health problems, I'm self-conscious and would rather not look sick, even if I know I am.

Nevertheless, I put my pride aside and walk into the gym feeling as if I have a bomb hidden underneath my clothes. I see a crowded weight room full of sweaty people, some of whom

I'm bound to know, so I find a spot in the least crowded area and try to avoid running into any familiar faces. Then, after a slow walk to a weight rack, I grab two twenty-pound dumbbells and lie in chest press position on a nearby bench. The dumbbells feel heavier than any weight I've ever lifted. My arms are unstable, shaking and swaying with every motor neuron misfire as I lift the weight directly above my face. I barely do three reps, then drop the dumbbells to the floor.

Suddenly I feel the Holter monitor slipping down my leg, followed by tension on my skin and then the unmistakable, jolting feeling of my unshaven chest hairs being yanked out. One of the electrodes connected to the Holter monitor has come unglued from my chest. I sit up and look around to see if anyone noticed, then reattach the electrode and shift the device back into place strapped on my thigh.

I continue to lift weights but feel increasingly sicker. My pain-riddled body won't stop throbbing. I'm preoccupied by the pain, but also hyper-aware of being exposed in my weakened state. I'm worried that one of my bodybuilding friends will see me and wonder why I'm lifting such light weight. Surely they would think I was joking and would insist that I join them for a more intense workout, which, at this point, would probably end me.

I need to get out of here. This is embarrassing. I'm too vulnerable, my status as a bodybuilder and fitness expert too compromised by my poor health and the weakness taking over my body. I don't think I can handle this much exertion right now, and I definitely can't afford to get any sicker. I'm exhausted and should be at home resting, tucked under the covers of my bed. I have fitness classes to teach and another semester of school to finish. If my health gets any worse, I won't be able to keep up with my busy schedule.

I'm terrified of getting sicker and losing control of my body. I've been in a constant state of fear that my health will continue to get worse, as if something is steadily sucking the life out of me and won't stop until there's nothing left, the thought of which is damn scary.

After leaving the gym, I get home and take a two-hour nap, then I find enough strength to return the Holter monitor to a local cardiologist, a colleague of Dr. Gretchen. He gives me a printout full of squiggly lines and says that, under the stress of exercise, my heart rhythms were normal. It doesn't make sense—every time I work out, my heart feels like it's going to explode, and the sound of it beating reverberates through my head. But the doctor assures me that the test is accurate and that my heart is healthy.

Now that I know this, I'm left wondering why exercise makes me so sick. This phenomenon is the furthest thing from what I've learned as a fitness instructor. I've been taught, as many people have, that exercise and physical activity should improve someone's health, not make it worse.

* * *

After returning home from seeing the cardiologist, I crawl into bed and take another nap. Final exams are over for the semester, and somehow, I've managed to pass all my classes, but now I'm too exhausted to celebrate. I may not have a choice though. Tonight Thomas and James are hosting a big Christmas party at our house.

When the party starts, I fill a cup with water and disguise it as vodka, then listlessly sip as I walk around the party. Mingling is draining and feels like a chore, but appearances must be maintained—the guests must see Healthy Jamison, not this sick version of him. Looking healthy is a big part of my job and I fear that if people know I'm sick, I'll lose credibility as a fitness instructor. But also, part of me believes that if I pretend to feel okay, eventually I will be.

A gulp of beer from Thomas's cup only adds to the feeling of wither and rot inside my body. The lights, sounds, and humidity of the party are wearing me down, penetrating my nerves with an intense sensory overload. Some friends have taken over my room, so I retreat to Thomas's room and lock the door. Lying on his musky bed, I close my eyes for a few minutes only to hear a knock on the door. I get up and open it. Molly's giddy smile appears, no doubt fueled by alcohol.

"Hey, cutie," she says, walking into the room. "Thomas told me you were in here hiding."

I close the door behind her. "Yeah, it's a little intense out there."

"No, it's not. You're just being lame," Molly says.

"Well, I just—"

"Hey, babe!" Molly interrupts me. "Babe, Baaa-be!"

"Yeah, what's up?" I say, as we stand next to Thomas's bed.

"I'm so glad you're feeling better now. You *are* better now, right?" she asks.

"Uh, I mean—"

"Yeah, you are. You're definitely feeling better," Molly says. "Look at you, all handsome and stuff. Babe, I really need you to sex me tonight."

"Oh, um," I stammer.

"You. Me. Sex. Right. Meow," she says, lifting up my shirt.

"Did you just say 'meow'?" I pull down my shirt. I'm not usually one to pass up sex, but I feel like shit, and I'm not in the mood. Plus it didn't go well last time, and I don't want to go through the embarrassment again.

"Maybe I did, maybe I didn't," Molly says. "That's for me to know and you to . . . not know." I give her a confused look, but she just smiles at me. "Hey, babe. Let's go to my place."

I know Molly wants to go to her house so we can have sex, and even though I'm not feeling up to it, I decide to go along, mostly so I can escape the loud party at my house.

On our way out the door, we dodge a gauntlet of people trying to get a ride home as we keep moving toward the Xterra parked outside. We get in and drive a few miles to Molly's place. As I climb the steps of the two-story townhouse, a flood of lactic acid hits my legs, and my lungs burn like I just hiked to the top of a tall mountain. Collapsing on Molly's bed is a relief, but one soon clouded by her sexual urgency. She pounces on me, pulls me off the bed, lifts my shirt, and kisses my chest. More sloppy kisses follow as I smell her warm alcohol-breath on my lips. Then she bites my neck, leaving a tender mark on my skin. It's the good kind of pain, not the caustic pain currently taking over the rest of my body while I try to get aroused.

I carry on the best I can. I should be resting, but I feel pressure from Molly, and myself, to have sex. It feels like an impossible task—I need to take off my clothes, and hers, while getting (and keeping) an erection as we continue our foreplay. We both have the same goal—pleasure—but it feels like the success of our love making, if we can even call it that, relies mostly on my ability to perform. And now, once again, I can't, not like this, not sick and with mounting pressure from my horny girlfriend.

The sick feeling inside my body tells me that it's all too much—the party, the car ride, the stairs, the foreplay, the sex. But how do I tell Molly that I need to stop and rest? She thinks I'm well when I'm obviously not. How do I not give her what she wants? How do I convince myself that it's okay to not have sex, to fail at this seemingly routine part of life?

In the end, I have no choice. My body expresses what my words cannot. I start to convulse—my legs and torso shake violently as I fall back on the bed. I have lost control. I try to surrender to the fragility of my body and the mercy of whatever is happening to it. My legs continue to shake as my limbs go numb and cold, and a wave of pain and nausea hits deep in my gut. In a near apoplectic state, my breaths are rapid and shallow. I try to slow my breathing and steady my heart rate, though all I really want to do is escape my body. I can't even escape my thoughts. Every bit of my focus is on the barrage of symptoms attacking me. I wish I could think about something else, anything other than how miserable I feel. I try to think of sandy beaches, scenic road trips, hot tubs, anything relaxing to distract myself from the siege of symptoms.

In the midst of the chaos, I have completely forgotten about Molly. I guess I hoped she would be checking on me by now, holding my hand and kissing my cheek. But perhaps she is too horrified by the tremors jolting through my body. I fear she will be traumatized by this health scare for months, if not years. I feel bad that I've put her through this. She shouldn't have to deal with this crap; she shouldn't have such an intimate, pleasurable experience tainted by my health problems.

I look across the bed to make sure Molly is okay. She's more than okay. She's asleep, comfortably resting on a pillow on the other side of the bed. Suddenly I don't feel bad for her anymore. But I do feel abandoned and angry that Molly seems not to care about my wellbeing. I know she's drunk and probably doesn't realize how sick I am, but fuck—she always does shit like this. She doesn't consider how her actions impact other people. One time we planned to go on a date, so I drove to her house, but when I got there, she told me that she was going to a bar with her friends instead. I was livid, but I pretended it was fine.

This time it's not fine. I'm done pretending that everything is okay. I'm not going to give Molly any more attention when I should be focusing on my health. It's hard to focus on anything, though, especially when I feel so alone, ashamed of my body, and frightened by the new depths of this illness. I want to be strong, like Keith and Tony, and all the other tough people I know, but something tells me that even they would be scared in this situation. So I let go of the façade, the virile persona I try so hard to present to everyone. Then I start to cry. Tears pour from the corners of my eyes and down the side of my face, like one of those Zen water fountains. I wail like an angry infant not knowing the significance of it all, not knowing the meaning of what's happening in my body. I can't remember the last time I cried like this. It was probably after the car accident, but that was a moment of grieving, this is a moment of fear and terror about what is happening inside my body. This is rock bottom. It must be; it can't possibly get worse.

I see Molly's cat curled up at the foot of the bed. He, too, is asleep and has somehow remained undisturbed throughout this whole episode. I'm the only one rattled in this bed, but I suppose that's for the best. Although, I do wish Molly were awake, holding me and whispering encouraging words in my ear while I wait for this scary moment to pass and my body to recover from the damage I've done to it.

CHAPTER 11

Tired of Being Tired

December 29, 2010

Yesterday I drove to my mom's house in Tuolumne, a small town in the heart of Gold Country at the foot of the Sierra Nevada. Once a home for miners, and later railroaders and loggers, now the streets of Tuolumne are nearly deserted, full of abandoned old buildings and defunct businesses. There are still some signs of life though, as a layer of smoke from wood stoves and burn piles settles over the tiny rural town.

I retreated here because I needed a break from my busy life. I'm too sick to work, exercise, and keep up with Molly. We've been drifting apart ever since she fell asleep during my tremor attack after the Christmas party. I woke up the next morning still feeling terrible, but she was oblivious to how I felt and everything that had happened the night before. Then she kept asking me to go to the gym and have dinner parties with her friends, and I just wasn't feeling up to any of it. So I'm taking a break from Molly and the rest of my life.

I've been in bed all day, tossing blankets and pillows around like a child caught in a nightmare. I'm trying to rest, but it feels like I'm just wasting time lying here. Being sick for this long has made me restless. Christmas has come and gone, and now the new year is only a few days away and I still feel as terrible as I did the first day I got sick at the gym.

Staying in Tuolumne with my mom, however temporarily, feels like an affront to my status as an independent adult. I've been fiercely independent my whole life, even as a child living with my mom. She'd take me to the store, and I'd buy my own groceries from a separate shopping cart. Once, when I was five, I even tried to drive our old Mazda sedan without her. I found my mom's keys and started the engine, but I couldn't see over the steering wheel and didn't know anything about a manual transmission, so the car lurched forward and took out the fence in our front yard.

I've always had a close, loving relationship with my mom, partly because she started respecting my autonomy at an early age, letting me do things my way or sometimes not at all. When I was four, she took me to my first day of swim lessons, and I refused to get in the pool. The instructor was very sweet, and all the other kids were having fun, but I still wouldn't get in the water. My mom was fine with it, though. She made sure that I had made up my mind, then she took me home, and I never went to another swim lesson. I may be a terrible swimmer now, but the fact that my mom respected my ability to make my own decisions back then has made me more self-sufficient as an adult.

That's why now it's so hard to let my mom take care of me. After three years of living on my own without my mom, I find myself relying on her for simple tasks, like cooking and doing laundry. I may be too sick to do those things for myself, but I need to do something. I'm tired of lying in bed, tired of the stagnation and ennui, tired of being tired for no reason. I've been in bed so long that lying here is no longer comfortable, and that's not to say that it was ever relaxing. There must only be a couple hours of daylight left, and I'm just now waking up, a casualty of lethargy.

I slowly sit up, my shoulders slouched as I try to rouse myself out of bed. Sunlight streams in through a nearby window, warming my face. I let the light wash over me as I stretch my limbs and feel a buzzing sensation under my legs. It's my phone vibrating on the bed. I look at the screen—a Sonoma County number is calling. I pick it up.

"Hello," a confident voice says on the other end of the phone. "Is Jamison Hill available?"

"This is Jamison."

"Hi, this is Dr. Gretchen. I have the results of your lab work," the doctor says. My stomach feels like an empty pit as nervousness takes over my body. I press the phone closer to my ear. "Based on your blood tests, it's clear that you have mononucleosis. As you know, I did a battery of tests, including the Holter monitor and a swab for strep throat, but those results all came back normal. However, the acute mono test, your elevated lymphocytes, and the test we did for the Epstein-Barr virus all indicate that you do in fact have mononucleosis."

"Oh," I say. I'm surprised and confused. Two weeks ago Dr. Gretchen told me that I was anxious and imagining my illness, but now she says I have mono. "So, does this mean it's not related to anxiety from my car accident?"

"Well, that's a good question." The doctor hesitates. "Psychological factors may still play a role, so I advise you to stay on the antidepressants. But it's safe to say that the main issue here is mononucleosis."

"Okay, so how do you treat it?" I ask.

"Unfortunately there is no treatment for mononucleosis. But don't worry, it's a very common illness," the doctor explains. "Most people get mononucleosis by the time they're an adult. Epstein-Barr virus, which causes the illness, will live in your body for the rest of your life, but eventually it will go dormant, all the symptoms will disappear, and you'll be back to normal." Dr. Gretchen pauses, breathing softly into the phone. "Jamison, I would like you to come in for a follow-up appointment in a few weeks, okay?"

"Okay, sure," I say.

"Great. Do you have any questions for me?" Dr. Gretchen asks.

"How long until I'm better?"

"I would say no longer than six weeks. Your energy should return as well. In the meantime, you may experience intense fatigue. It can be extreme—some people can't do simple errands like shop for groceries. So for now just rest as much as you can, and because your spleen is enlarged, no tackle football."

How about heavy squats? Or flipping a tractor tire with a weighted vest on? Ask her if you can still do three-hour workouts and eat under two thousand calories a day.

Dr. Gretchen tells me that most, if not all, of my symptoms are fairly typical for mononucleosis. The weakness, the chills, the swollen lymph nodes, the muscle pain, and the brain fog are all part of the illness. Everything I've been experiencing makes sense now. I resist the urge to jump out of bed and do a back flip, or some plyometric push-ups. Instead I throw my fists in the air and do a short sparring session with the blankets and pillows before wearing myself out. I'm exhausted but I don't care; any fatigue I feel now will be gone in a matter of weeks. I can feel the helplessness and frustration melting away already. It's only a matter of time until I'm able to resume life as I know it. It's already been a month, a couple more weeks and

I should be ready for school to start again, ready to get back to working and lifting weights like this illness never happened.

Feeling hopeful about my new prognosis, I call Jaron, who runs the group fitness company I work for, and tell him that I'm sick and can't make it to the next boot camp. Thankfully he says he'll teach the class for a couple weeks while I recover. It's a relief that Jaron is so understanding. Over the last year, he has become my mentor, teaching me the many facets of the fitness industry. I'm excited to get back to work with him in the new year.

Once I'm off the phone with Jaron, I get dressed and see a movie with my mom and my sister, Claire, who lives in the Santa Cruz Mountains, about sixty miles south of San Francisco. Like me, Claire has come to Tuolumne to visit my mom for the holidays.

She's eight years older than me, but despite our age difference, we've always had a presence in each other's lives. I haven't seen her in several months because I've been busy with school and work, but when I was a little kid, we spent a lot of time together. She'd always let me hang out and wrestle with her friends, or she'd take me on joy rides through the mountains. We'd drive around for hours, listening to the same 90s pop songs on the stereo. As we've grown older and become adults, it's been hard to keep in touch at times—she's moved around a lot, and I've gone away to college—but we always reunite at my mom's house at least a couple times a year.

This time our reunion is at the movie theater. But the loud audio and large screen is wearing me down, making me tired and filling my muscles and joints with pain. I try to wait until the symptoms pass, but the only relief I find is in knowing that soon the exhaustion and other symptoms will be gone, a small blip in my otherwise healthy life.

After the movie, we stop at a sushi restaurant. The hostess shows us to a table, and we sit down. I look across the table at my mom, her short brown hair ruffling around as she takes off her coat. Claire is sitting next to me, bundled up in a black jacket and matching beanie.

Within a few minutes, I feel extremely fatigued and overwhelmed by everything in the restaurant—the florescent lighting burning my eyes, the competitive chatter buzzing in my ears, and the rising heat flaring up my symptoms.

I excuse myself from the table and make my way to the entrance of the restaurant while trying to avoid the bomb of energy in the room threatening to swallow up what's left of my strength. My arms are weak, and I have to use most of my body weight as leverage to push open the entrance door.

I finally make it outside and sit on the cold concrete curb. I've only been out of bed a couple hours, and I'm already spent, my body consumed by immense fatigue. It feels like I just ran a hundred-mile race and was hit by a large truck in the final stretch.

I bow my head in my hands and take a deep breath. There's something about moments like this, moments of utter helplessness, that leave me wanting to escape, looking for a break from the chaos surrounding me and the pain inside me. That, and I always seem to embrace cold, blemished concrete in these moments, as I did that day on the Napa River Bridge.

For a long time I just sit on the curb, repeatedly telling myself that this will all be over soon. I will get better. I have to get better. Dr. Gretchen said I will.

CHAPTER 12

Two Ways of Life Converge

January 31, 2011

The night sky is dark and ominous, covered with a thick layer of smoke settling over my mom's house in Tuolumne. I'm about to drive back to Sonoma County with my belongings packed into a large laundry hamper—everything from toiletries and shoes to Christmas gifts and my laptop are crammed in the hamper like a bunch of junk on its way to the thrift store.

On my way to the car, my phone buzzes with a voicemail from Jaron. He's making sure I'll be teaching my boot camp class tomorrow evening. I send him a confirmation text, then get in the driver's seat, holding the door open for my mom to say goodbye, her soft features tightening with worry as she gives me a hug.

"Are you sure you're up for this, kiddo?" she asks.

"I have to go for it, Mom. School and boot camp aren't going to wait."

"Okay, but don't push yourself too hard. Know your limits. And please call if you need me," she says, giving me another hug and closing the car door.

The roads in the Central Valley are without streetlamps for much of the first half of the drive. Around Manteca the lights of civilization finally come out to play. Then I pass Tracy, a city surrounded by farmland and seemingly endless rows of shopping malls and suburban housing developments. Eventually I make it to the bright city lights of Oakland and San Francisco, the mechanical sounds of public transportation whirring along the multi-lane freeway. It's a stark contrast to the dark, quiet atmosphere back in Tuolumne. The lights along the freeway are brighter, the sounds are louder, and the air is, well, surprisingly fresher than the smoke from the smoldering burn piles around my mom's house.

Finally I pull into my driveway on Mary Place, ready to soak up the familiarity of being back home. Inside the house, James and Thomas are in the middle of an intense video game session, but they pause when they see me standing in the doorway, smiling at them. It's good to see them, good to be home, a relief, really. Being sick and staying with my mom made me worry that I'd have to give up my autonomy, that I'd have to let go of my life in Sonoma and move to Tuolumne permanently. Now I just have to be well enough to stay here and take care of myself.

After some hugs and fist bumps, I talk to Thomas and James for a few minutes, each of us recapping our respective holidays. Then I unload my laundry hamper from the Xterra and check my phone. It's about ten thirty. I'm exhausted, but the excitement from being home and seeing my friends keeps me on my feet long enough to do my laundry. Then, finally, I collapse on my bed and fall asleep.

CHAPTER 13

Sixty Seconds Feel Like Sixty Minutes

February 1 – 2, 2011

It's Tuesday morning, and I'm lying in bed after getting home from a visit to Dr. Gretchen's office. The six-week mark has passed, and I still feel like shit. Dr. Gretchen told me that some cases of mono last longer than expected and because there's no treatment for the illness, all I can do is wait for the Epstein-Barr virus to run its course. The doctor didn't say much else or offer insight about when or how I'll recover, only that I should make another appointment with her in a few months if I'm not feeling better.

It made me angry how dismissive and apathetic she was about something that has taken over my life. And now she gets to move on and go about her job, dismissing patients without any consequences. It makes me want to send her a huge box of dog shit and watch her open it just so she can experience a tiny bit of the turmoil that I've been through.

As much as I want to pass my anger on to Dr. Gretchen, I'm not going to. Instead, for the time being, I'm going to figure out how to live with this stupid illness. I'm not exactly sure what that means or how long it'll last; I just know that it's my only choice.

Now I'm resting for the day ahead, trying not to think about all the obligations I've made that I won't be able to fulfill. A few weeks ago, I registered for eight hours of classes on Tuesdays and Thursdays this semester. It's the only way I can finish my remaining units and graduate with my friends in a few months.

To make things worse, I also committed to teaching boot camp class every weekday evening and weekend morning. I knew it was an ambitious schedule but thought I'd be better by now and able to handle it. Now it's daunting to even think about getting myself to class and work. The enormity of the situation is weighing on me, and so is the impossible task of trying to figure out what I'm capable of accomplishing today.

You know exactly what you're capable of accomplishing today, and it's less, way less, than what you have planned. You can't sit through eight hours of class feeling like this. Even a healthy person would struggle taking that many classes.

What's left of my optimism fades, and I decide to reduce my schedule and not go to my classes today. Instead I lie on my flattened, drool-stained pillow and close my eyes. My plan is to stay in bed long enough, the entire day if necessary, so I have enough energy to teach my boot camp class tonight. Jaron has already filled in for me the last several weeks, and I'm afraid that if I don't show up tonight, he'll fire me. If I can eke out an appearance at boot camp, then maybe I can parlay that into making it to some of my classes on Thursday. That is, after convincing my professors to grant me amnesty for missing the first day of class.

While I remain in bed, nausea and hunger team against me like a pair of evil villains riddling my mind and torturing my body. I need to eat something, but there isn't much food in the kitchen. I could go to the grocery store, but that would take every bit of energy I have, leaving me none to teach boot camp class. Being this debilitated and hungry gives me a primal fear, however irrationally, that I'm going to starve, a fear that prompts me to use precious energy to walk to the kitchen. There I find a carton of egg whites in the refrigerator. I pour the viscous liquid into a bowl and cook it in the microwave, then return to bed with a plate full of the bland eggs and a few raw almonds, the only food I had in the pantry. The meal gives me some nourishment, but mostly just makes me want to vomit.

Needing a distraction from the virulent sickness inside my body, I find a house remodeling show on TV. But the sensory stimulation from the large screen rattles my nerves and makes my brain feel like its short circuiting, the way a computer shuts off and reboots itself when there's a problem. I try watching a movie on my laptop, but it proves just as difficult to tolerate; so does playing a game on my phone. This sensory overload is exertion at its lowest point—energy I've never considered significant, if at all. The only thing left for me to do is stare at the contents of my room like a visitor in a museum, looking without touching.

After several hours in bed, unable to sleep, I start to panic. There's only about forty minutes before I need to be at boot camp, and I don't feel any better. Teaching a group fitness class when I can barely take care of myself seems impossible and incredibly foolish, but I take a deep breath and decide to do it anyway.

On the way to the class in Santa Rosa, I take a detour to Jaron's house to pick up the new client roster. With the car accident and my illness looming in my mind, driving doesn't feel entirely safe—the vertigo makes it feel like the road is crumbling beneath my car. I drive slowly and stay alert, but it does little to assuage my fears. I'm only a few blocks from my house, and I already want to go home. I could turn around and be back in bed in five minutes. But I can't do that to myself. I can't let this illness take my job, the only one I've ever loved.

My knuckles tap on the hard surface of Jaron's double front doors with rectangular recessed paneling that I've never noticed before, or maybe in my disoriented state I just forgot it was there. Jaron opens one of the doors, and I put on my best healthy-person face, but I can feel the façade slipping. My vertigo distorts everything I see—Jaron's short, stocky figure looks tall and distant, like I'm peering through the wrong end of binoculars. He welcomes me inside, and the walls start swirling around me, like the house is spinning and I'm its axis. I try to ignore it and focus on Jaron as he busily moves around his home office, shuffling papers and telling me about all the things he's done today. As we talk, he multitasks like healthy, energetic people do, but I just sit slumped over in an old, creaky chair, my eyes shifting around, trying to follow his movements. I'm amazed at how I've spent the entire day in bed just to have a chance at completing one hour of work—a mere fraction of Jaron's day.

By the time I arrive at boot camp class, the pain and weakness are in full force. But I have to push through it. I have to teach this class. Greeting my clients is a challenge—it takes all my concentration just to give them some semblance of a smile. Thankfully none of them heckle me today, a minor miracle considering they still have no idea that I'm sick, no idea that I barely made it here.

Once class begins, I demonstrate some plyometric squats and my body reacts with vengeance. The pain is stabbing at my legs, and I'm so dizzy it feels like I could pass out and smack my head on the pavement at any moment. The next half hour goes by at a glacial pace as I give my clients several long water breaks so I can rest. Then, when I can barely stand anymore, I end class twenty minutes early and slowly shuffle back to my car.

On the way home, I make a quick stop at a drive-thru to order something more palatable than almonds and egg whites. I rarely eat fast food, but I'm desperate for sustenance and want to get back to the comfort of my bed as soon as possible.

Back at my house, the sick feeling intensifies as I lie in my unmade bed, waiting for time to pass, hoping my reality isn't real and the truth of the situation isn't true. I stare motionless at the ceiling of my room, shadows casting over me in the darkened space as I huddle under my comforter and three layers of clothing, regretting that I've pushed my body this far. The only thing I can do is brace for oncoming symptoms, and there are lots of them. The tremors are back, shooting through my body like electrical shocks. The nausea and vertigo aren't helping either, and the pain filling every part of my body is nearly unbearable.

The symptoms are so bad that time feels like it's slowing down—sixty seconds feel like sixty minutes. I've been listening to an *Oliver Twist* audiobook on my phone to distract myself, and it almost works. The narrator's British accent is soothing, giving me a little bit of comfort amid the fury of aggressive symptoms. But it fails to make me forget how sick I feel.

In the thick of it, I try to keep my thoughts positive, but the best I can do is imagine my antibodies fighting the Epstein-Barr virus, the thought of which reminds me of an old picture book about Louis Pasteur's rabies vaccine that I used to flip through as a kid. It depicted a boy bit by a rabid dog, then toy soldiers symbolizing the vaccine charged in and killed the rabies. The battle in my body isn't going as well. My antibodies aren't working. I need my own toy soldiers to venture in and destroy the virus. I need, so badly, to be done with this illness.

* * *

It's the middle of the night, and my condition has gotten worse. I had to stop listening to *Oliver Twist* because my head is pounding with pressure, and I'm too disoriented to concentrate on anything. The physical consequences of teaching boot camp have caught up with me—pain is pulsing throughout my body amid a surge of weakness paralyzing my muscles, and the tremors are shaking my metal bed frame like a violent earthquake.

It seems nearly certain that I won't be well enough to go to my classes on Thursday, which means I'll have to drop out of school for the semester. But I've never dropped out of school before, and giving up on something that important makes me worry about my future. In search of guidance and comfort, I call my mom for the third time in the last few hours.

"Hey kiddo, how are you feeling?" She sounds tired and concerned.

"Not good," I say. "It hasn't gotten any better."

"Why don't you let me come get you?" she asks.

"It's a four-hour drive." My voice is worn and raspy.

"That doesn't matter. You need someone to help you."

"But I don't want to drop out of school and lose my job."

"Sweetie, you have to be honest with yourself about the situation," my mom says. "You are very sick, which means you may need to give up some parts of your life until you recover."

"That's . . ." My voice cracks. I can feel my eyes brim with tears. "That's not what I want to hear. If I fight hard enough, I always get through it. I've never had to give up like this."

"I know, but you may not have a choice right now, and in your case, not giving up may mean recuperating and taking care of yourself," my mom says. "Your body is trying to tell you something. It needs rest."

"Rest? I've spent more time resting in the last two months than I have in the last two years. How much more rest do I need?" I prop myself up in the corner of my bed, my chest heaving as tears lug down my face and tremors rattle my legs.

"It's frustrating, I know, but you need as much rest as it takes to get better," my mom says. I sniffle and blow a frustrated breath into the phone. "You really don't sound good. Will you please let me come get you?"

"I don't know, Mom."

"You can rest up at my house, and I can always bring you back when you start feeling better."

"All right, I guess."

"Good," she says. "I'll see you in a few hours. Try to get some sleep."

CHAPTER 14

Low and Growly

February 24, 2011

Each step feels like a risk, each movement makes me wonder if personal hygiene is worth the effort, if taking a shower is really worth making myself feel worse. Ultimately, I decide that yes, I must take a shower because I haven't bathed in several days and I smell like shit.

I grip and re-grip the cold, slightly greasy stairway railing as I ascend the steps to the bathroom. It feels like I'm bracing for the end of the world, or maybe just the end of mine. At the top of the stairs I get dizzy, lose my balance, and fall to my knees. My lungs burn, and I gasp for air. After a couple minutes of catching my breath, I get to my feet, hobble to the bathroom, and turn on the light. It stings my eyes, so I flip it off. Then I put in earplugs to block out the loud sound of the water hitting the bathtub as I run the faucet. I wait until the water is warm, then I step into the tub, putting my weight against the shower wall. My legs are weak and tired, trembling as they struggle to hold up the rest of my body.

I consider putting a chair in the shower, but I refuse to abuse my ego in such a way. Not to mention, I'm too weak to carry a chair upstairs, and I don't want to ask my mom for help. The most logical thing would be for me to just lie in the tub and soak, but I prefer the shower and taking a bath just seems like an admission of defeat.

The water from the shower cascades down my back as gravity weakens my stance—even my lean five-foot-eight, one-hundred-sixty-pound body is too heavy for my ailing muscles. I fall to one knee, then both, and finally plop down in the middle of the tub while the warm water blasts my head. I want to stand up, but it's pointless. There's nobody to impress by standing, not even myself. Sitting in the tub is freeing—my muscles can relax. But my mind is still focused on the sickness inside my body and how my life has unraveled over the last few months.

I think of the morning my mom drove to Rohnert Park to take me back to Tuolumne, the morning after I was supposed to start my last semester of college but couldn't. I was too weak to walk, and my one-hundred-ten-pound, fifty-year-old mother had to practically carry me to the car. Since then, I've asked her to sleep in my bed with me for comfort while the sickness and viral battle rages in my body. It makes me feel like a scared child. Every night my mom tells me that I'm going to get better, that I just need to find peace with the illness until I do. Then she reads me a book before lying down and falling asleep next to me as I remain awake, riding out the waves of symptoms.

After drying off and putting on clothes, I try to walk downstairs, but my legs quickly give out, so I sit on the steps and slide down them on my ass one at a time. It takes several minutes, but eventually I make it to the bottom floor. Then I crawl into my makeshift bed—a pull-out couch in my mom's living room.

As a distraction, I watch Jack LaLanne workout videos from the 1950s on my phone. They are relics from a simpler time long before I was born, but they possess a nostalgic quality that I enjoy. Jack spouts off his workout wisdom to the 1950s viewer, and to me—an admirer from the future, one too weak to do even his simplest exercises. That's not entirely true though, I can do his face exercises, comical mouth contortions that require little energy, but I guess they still count for something.

My face workout is soon interrupted by my phone vibrating. It's Molly calling. We haven't seen or spoken to each other much since the Christmas party, and now that school has started and I'm not in Sonoma, I suspect she will want to move on with her life.

I put the phone to my ear. "Hi," Molly says. "When are you coming back?"

"I don't know. Hopefully soon," I say.

"What are you waiting for?" she asks, her tone snippy.

"Well, I'm still sick. I had to give up teaching boot camp, and it looks like I'm not going to graduate on time."

"Oh, but are you really that sick?" Molly asks.

"What do you mean? I wouldn't give all that up for nothing."

"But you seemed fine the last time I saw you," she says. "I mean, you didn't even look sick."

"Well, I *was* sick, and I still am." My voice is low and growly.

"You're just being a downer. Maybe that doctor was right, you could just be depressed." I want to tell Molly to stop judging me, but before I can say anything, I hear rustling and people talking to her on the other end of the phone. "Oh hey, I gotta go," she says. "Call me when you're back in town."

We hang up and I get a feeling that our relationship is over. I can tell, however tacitly, that Molly doesn't genuinely want me to call her unless I'm feeling better. She wants Healthy Jamison to call her. She wants the ripped guy from the gym who used to go jogging with her. She wants the guy who drove to her house every night to have sex, not the guy who needs someone to take care of him. She doesn't want Sick Jamison. She doesn't even think I'm sick. And I resent her for it. I resent her for a lot of things. I've needed Molly's help over the last several weeks, and she hasn't been there for me. She couldn't even stay awake while I was having a tremor attack when we tried to have sex after the Christmas party.

Since the beginning, our relationship has revolved around two things—sex and working out—and now that I can't do either, the shallow nature of our connection has been exposed and the relationship has collapsed. But I'm not going to feel bad about it. I'm not going to give any more of my energy to her. I'm just going to move on.

CHAPTER 15

Five Hundred Feet of Pavement Pounding

April 17, 2011

In the past month, I've managed to regain some of my health. I still can't go back to work or school, but I do feel a bit better, well enough to go for a walk today, maybe even a little run. But first I need to find the right place—ideally somewhere secluded where no one will see me look sick and weak as I try to rehabilitate my body.

Buchanan Road, a winding street following a steep river gorge just outside of Tuolumne, is a good spot. Bright sunlight hits the front of the car as I find a turnoff with a sprawling view of the Stanislaus National Forest. Here, on the seal coated asphalt overlooking the Tuolumne River streaming through seemingly endless lines of pine trees, is where I will try to exercise.

Whether I'm indeed able to exercise is uncertain, but just being out of the house is an accomplishment. It feels rejuvenating but foreign, like visiting an unfamiliar country—exciting and a little scary. I can handle these feelings, but the discontent about my body's deconditioning is much harder to live with, which is why I've decided to torture myself with exercise today. Hopefully I don't overdo it, but I probably will. I've never been good at light exercise. It feels impossible, especially in this moment, to not push myself past my limits.

The smart thing to do would be to simply walk along the gravelly pavement for a few minutes, then turn around and go home. Given my condition, that would probably be the right amount of exercise. But I know it won't be enough for me. I have to at least try to run. If all I'm going to do is walk, I might as well turn around right now. For me, walking isn't a workout; it's a leisure activity. Walking was what I did to get to the gym. It was my transportation, my warmup, not the workout itself. As stubborn as that may seem, it's the foundation for my inner drive and self-discipline, the fuel I used to work out every day. Then I got sick and it became more than that. It helped me get through some truly scary moments lying in bed, unsure of what was happening inside my body. Now I hope it will propel me forward, so I can fully recover from this illness and get my life back.

When I look up from the asphalt, I see lush green trees lining the surrounding mountain ridges. My shoes tap the gravel, setting off a storm of stiffness in my bones and weakness in my muscles. It's unpleasant, but that's okay. I just want to run a little, or at least move at a pace faster than when I walk from my bed to the bathroom each morning.

Preparing for this run makes me miss working out. I miss the pre-workout ritual of getting dressed, eating, taking supplements, grabbing my gear, and hitting the road. I miss lifting weights, throwing dumbbells around the gym like a child in a room full of toys. I miss running—pumping my arms and legs, creating my own wind. I even miss the misshapen wear marks on my shoes.

Starting with a slow walk, I keep my eyes forward, bracing myself to bump up the pace. But my body gets weaker the more it moves and pain shoots through my thighs, then up my back. Without warning, my muscles make a disproportionate exchange of ATP for inflammation, and the pain gets worse. I'm not even jogging yet, and I'm already about to fall over. If I wait any longer to run, I may have nothing left. So I go all out, picking my feet up and sprinting down the pavement. It's not the smartest decision, especially for my body, but I don't care. It brings me joy, and a few seconds of normalcy, a tiny glimpse of how my life had been before this illness.

I make it about five hundred feet before the symptoms are too strong to continue. My pace grinds to a stop, and I feel like I'm going to pass out. I take a few seconds to find my equilibrium, then turn around and look down the road at my car. I had hoped the Xterra would be out of sight by now, but there it is, still in my view.

Slowly, painfully, I walk back to the car. My lungs are burning and wheezing, my joints and muscles protesting each step I take. But there is also something new—a new symptom, an odd pricking sensation poking at my skin. It would have freaked me out when I first got sick, but now I know it's just another mysterious symptom, like the bevy of others that will almost certainly leave me holed up in bed recuperating from this short run.

At some point in the next several days, I will likely ask myself if five hundred feet of pavement-pounding, arm-pumping, wind-on-my-face exercise was worth it, worth the recovery—the pain and immobility, the monotonous lying in bed staring at the ceiling, worth the incessant boredom and the frustration of needing my mom to take care of me. Then, after I'm done hating myself for such a simple and justifiable act, I will conclude that yes, absolutely, it was worth it, because sometimes I just need to swear off what's best for this ailing body of mine and do what makes me happy.

CHAPTER 16

Jaws of Life

May 1, 2011

Once again, I'm driving from Tuolumne back to my house in Sonoma. My mom's tailing me in her yellow Volkswagen Beetle, acting as a safety net in case I can't drive myself the entire way. That would be a nightmare—I'd have to leave my car on the side of the road miles from my house—but at this point, it's a definite possibility.

I'm feeling weak and sick to my stomach, two things that don't mix well with driving. And the cars speeding past me on the highway make it worse. I'm nervous that one of them will clip my bumper and send me fishtailing across the highway, crashing into other cars before rolling into a ditch, where the Xterra will lie mangled, and the paramedics will have to use the Jaws of Life to rescue me. It's a thought hard to shake off, especially when I'm feeling sick, but in some ways the illness is a distraction and makes thoughts of the car accident easier to dismiss.

It helps that the laminated hospital bracelet is still pinned to the overhead visor above my head. The adhesive is almost gone, and the lamination is coming undone as time wears on it, but I'm not ready to get rid of it, not ready to give up my totem and the symbolism it holds.

I am ready to move on with my life and recover from this illness though. I need to get back to work. Jaron has hired another fitness instructor to teach my boot camp class, but he said I can return to work as soon as I'm feeling well enough. I also need to finish school. My friends will be graduating without me in a few weeks, but I can still complete my degree next semester. These are parts of my life that can be repaired as my health returns. But first, before I can do anything, I need to get back home safely.

After more than three hours of driving, the most I've done since December, I pull into my driveway on Mary Place and check my phone. It's about four in the afternoon, but my weary body makes it feel like three in the morning. Driving has taken an immense toll on me. I need a long, flat, and ideally soft surface to lie on.

Once I push aside the stack of mail piled in front of my bedroom door, I walk into five-month-old stale air and a mess straight out of an episode of *Hoarders*. There's dust everywhere, on everything. Pillows and protein bar wrappers are scattered on the floor. My comforter is clumped into a ball in the corner of my bed, and my closet door is wide open. I resist the urge to clean and instead do what is best for my health: nothing.

I lie in my unmade bed and close my eyes, but before I put my problems away with a dream, my mom comes in to check on me.

"Hey, kiddo. Can I get you anything?" she asks, sitting on the edge of my bed.

"I'm all right, thanks," I say, grabbing her hand and giving it a squeeze.

"I'm going to stick around for a bit to make sure you're okay here on your own."

"Thanks, Mom. I need to find a way to stay here and take care of myself. I'm just worried that I won't be able to keep up with Thomas and James." I let out a long sigh. "Going to bed at nine every night doesn't really mesh with the college lifestyle."

"Don't worry about that. Just make sure James and Thomas know what is going on with you, and let the rest take care of itself," my mom says, kissing me on the forehead and leaving me to rest.

CHAPTER 17

Little Liquid Missiles

May 28, 2011

Thomas walks in the front door. It looks as if his steps are insulated by air as he moves through the house carrying a neatly folded cap and gown. Sonoma State's graduation is today, and many of my friends, including Thomas and Kendra, will be walking in the ceremony. I will not, thanks to the four classes I still need to finish.

Thomas asks if I'm going to watch the graduation ceremony, and immediately I feel guilty for not wanting to go. I politely tell him that I can't make it. But the truth is, I don't want to be there because I'm jealous, full of envy and frustration that he's graduating and I'm not. In a few hours he'll be achieving something that I was so close to accomplishing myself. It feels like we were running a race, neck-and-neck, and then in the final stretch, I stepped in a ditch, broke my ankle, and had to watch as Thomas crossed the finish line without me.

Instead of sitting around feeling sorry for myself, I get up and find the Univega leaning against a wall in the garage. The old, metallic blue bike has flat tires and it's covered in spiderwebs. Now it looks more like a mangy shelter dog than a faithful Labrador wagging its tail for a walk. But I can fix that. I think. Inflating the tires and dusting off the frame siphons much of my energy. I don't care though; this bike ride is happening regardless of how bad I feel. Any caution or logic that I have about not pushing myself too much is erased by my stubborn need to exercise.

It begins to rain while I hop on the Univega and pedal down the street, a sudden rush of joy massaging my soul as my blood pumps faster. It's a good feeling, but a distant one, like a childhood memory. I cruise by the rhythmic rallying of tennis balls across the street from my house and turn right onto Bodway, the Univega's tires treading over the slick asphalt. My muscles start to feel the effects of pedaling as nausea creeps into my stomach, and I'm getting more disoriented by the second.

The rain is now shooting down from the dark clouds above like little liquid missiles landing on me and drizzling off my fingers gripping the Univega's curved handlebars. My black mesh jacket and sweatpants are absolutely soaked and splattered with mud from the dirty road.

A few miles in the opposite direction, everyone at the graduation ceremony is probably just as wet and muddy. Part of me, the better part, wishes I were there, watching Thomas achieve a huge milestone in his life. I owe him that. I owe him for checking on me when I first got sick, for all the times he's made me food when I wasn't well enough to make it myself. I wish I could put aside my bitterness and just be happy for my friend instead of selfishly skipping the ceremony to take out my frustrations on a bike ride. But, for better or worse, that's what I've chosen to do.

I pedal faster to get away from the graduation, away from my inadequacies and regrets, away from the rain and under the shelter of trees canopying the road. But the shelter quickly disappears, and the surroundings transition from suburban houses to open farmland as the rain gets thicker and more violent, blasting me in the face.

Bodway comes to a dead end, so I pump the brakes and pull the Univega off the road. If I turn left, I can continue on, but with the rain coming down harder and my weakened muscles throbbing, that would be a bad idea. Despite my reckless state of mind and urge to keep going, I make the wise decision to turn around and pedal home. Turning back is the smart choice, one I don't like making but will have to live with. Though it may not make a difference—I'll probably still suffer the consequences of this short burst of exertion, as I did last month when I tried to go for a run in Tuolumne.

By the time I get home, the nausea is so bad that I head straight for the bathroom. I dry heave over the toilet for a few minutes, then sit on the cold tile floor and catch my breath. My muscles are weak, and my body hurts all over. The fatigue I feel is similar to the feeling I used to get the day after one of my three-hour workouts, except this feeling is more intense and more immediate, and all I did was cruise around on my bike for a few minutes.

My workouts used to give me a sense of calm and a rush of endorphins, but now they just make me feel miserable. Every time I try to exercise, I feel significantly worse. And this time is no exception.

While gingerly sprawling out on the couch, I wonder how long it will take me to recover from this act of defiance against the illness plaguing my body. I suspect it will be somewhere in the range of three to five days before I get back to my baseline, a decent guess based on past experiences. The usual symptoms—nausea, exhaustion, pain, and weakness—will likely come on strong, as they've already started to, hitting hard with flu-like strength. By day three or five, the symptoms will lessen, then a subtle amount of energy will creep back into my body. A manageable level of the illness will then persist until, once again, I decide to torture myself with exercise.

CHAPTER 18

An Illness With a Shitty Name

June 7, 2011

During a recent appointment with Dr. Gretchen, I told her that my health has improved some, but I still struggle with many of the same symptoms, especially pain, nausea, and fatigue. I still feel like I'm going to puke or pass out every time I try to exercise, but the doctor offered little help.

I asked her if I still have mononucleosis, or if something else is afflicting me. She said that a patient who has mono or severe fatigue that lasts longer than six months can be diagnosed with an illness called chronic fatigue syndrome, which sounds like something doctors use to diagnose people who don't fit the mold of any other illness. It also sounds like a single-symptom illness, but I have a myriad of symptoms other than fatigue.

Nonetheless, Dr. Gretchen still diagnosed me with chronic fatigue syndrome. According to her, there's no diagnostic test for CFS, but there is additional criteria that can be applied to diagnose patients with the illness, mostly "nonspecific" symptoms like feeling unwell for more than twenty-four hours after physical exertion, muscle pain, memory issues, headaches, joint pain, sleep problems, and tender lymph nodes—all of which I have.

Dr. Gretchen told me there is no cure for CFS, or even an effective treatment. Although she did prescribe me more antidepressants, which must mean she still thinks my illness is psychological, caused by residual trauma from my car accident.

Maybe it's a defense mechanism—maybe she gives "happy pills" to all her patients with tough cases, maybe she doesn't know what else to do. The antidepressants obviously don't work for you because your illness isn't depression; it's not in your head nor is it caused by the trauma from the car accident. It's knocking you on your ass every time you try to work out or do anything physical. You can't even go to the grocery store without feeling worse. And the nausea—oh, the fucking nausea—leaves you in a fetal position wrapped around the toilet every night. These things are physical, not imagined or caused by anxiety and depression.

Before I left her office, Dr. Gretchen told me to see a CFS specialist. But when I asked her for a referral, she said she didn't know of any doctors who specialize in the illness. So until I find one, I'm on my own, stuck with a broken body, fighting an illness with a shitty name, one I didn't even know existed until recently.

CHAPTER 19

Sandpaper on Bare Skin Rough

September 18, 2011

Finding a doctor who specializes in chronic fatigue syndrome is proving to be difficult. After searching online, asking several doctors for referrals, and even looking in the phone book without success, I started to think, however absurdly, that Dr. Gretchen was messing with me. I thought maybe she was playing a cruel joke wherein she diagnoses unsuspecting patients with a made-up illness and gives it a condescending name like wimpy cough disorder or, in my case, chronic fatigue syndrome. But the other doctors I talked to knew of CFS and said it is in fact a real illness. Unfortunately, none of them have enough expertise to treat me, so for now, I've decided to put my search for a specialist on hold and focus on finishing my degree.

The fall semester has started at Sonoma State, and the first week of class was rough, sandpaper on bare skin rough. Just like last semester, I tried to take four classes, but the schedule quickly overwhelmed me. I was able to make it to the first day, but my body didn't do well, and once again a full schedule was too ambitious for me while battling the illness. Though I did manage to salvage the semester by taking the minimum—one class.

It feels frivolous to accept an extra seven thousand dollars in student loan debt just to take one class, but without it, I couldn't pay my rent and would have to go back to Tuolumne and live with my mom. Staying at Sonoma State and finishing my courses at the slowest pace possible is expensive, maybe even a luxury given my privilege in this world, but it's also crucial to my autonomy and getting back on my feet.

My first, and only, class of the semester is a leadership course, and it's not going to be easy. The professor assigned a presentation about leadership styles depicted in popular movies like *Saving Private Ryan*. It's due in a few weeks, and I'm a little nervous about getting up in front of the class. Though I doubt it will be as intimidating as, say, posing nearly naked in front of hundreds of people at a bodybuilding competition. Mostly I'm nervous about how my body will handle standing upright for twenty minutes during the presentation. I suspect it will be hard for me to stay on my feet that long—my muscles will probably struggle to support my body weight—but if I'm strategic and pace myself, I know I can get through it.

Luckily it's a group presentation, so the entire workload won't fall on me. But it still comes with a lot of pressure. If I'm unable to do the presentation, I'll fail the class, and all my efforts will be wasted. I'm betting everything—my health and my recovery—on being able to pass this class. It's either that or let the illness completely consume my life, and that's just not an option.

Other than being assigned the group presentation, my first day in class was fairly routine. It felt as though everything had remained the same, except me. Many of my friends were still on campus, their lives unchanged since the last time I saw them. My life had changed, though.

My body especially had gone through a drastic transformation, and some of my classmates noticed. A few of them commented on how much weight I had lost. I was, of course, too proud to tell them it was because I'm sick. Pretending to be oblivious to my body's deterioration was easier than telling the truth, and I wanted my classmates to believe that I was still healthy, or at least not ill. I think I did a convincing job too. After all, there I was back in action, walking, talking, even smiling, as if I were fine, as if nothing had happened.

I'm not sure how, but I've developed this ability to function reasonably well and make myself seem healthy while I've been sick. I look normal, but most people never see me on days when I'm too sick to get out of bed. For me, and I suspect many people who have "invisible" illnesses like mine, the innate ability to act healthy doesn't make being sick any easier—quite the opposite, in fact. It makes life more difficult, but the last thing I want is pity or someone catering to me because I'm sick. Not to mention, trying to describe my illness to a classmate, or anyone really, is about as frustrating as a conversation gets, and I find a feeble explanation too easily sounds like complaining, or worse, hypochondria. So I resolve to let my classmates think I'm as healthy as I was a year ago. It's simpler that way, even though in many ways it's not. It's how I keep the illness from completely taking over my life and from destroying the image of myself as a virile bodybuilder, which I've worked so hard to create.

I'm determined to go the entire semester without my class-mates knowing about my illness, or the precautions I have to take just to get to class, just to be on par with them for two hours twice a week. While I exert as little energy as possible—either recovering from, or preparing for, each day—my classmates are off playing frisbee at the park or grabbing a bite to eat. I, on the other hand, sit on the couch—my eyes closed and my body still—meditating on the sickness inside me and how I'm lucky to accomplish a single task before my energy envelope is torn wide open.

My friends in class know me as a bodybuilder, not as a sick person, which is what I want, but under the circumstances, it's a difficult illusion to maintain. Because they don't know that I'm sick, and my body isn't in the shape it once was, they probably think that I've gotten lazy and stopped working out. Perhaps that's why they talk about how my body has changed. Their words are unintentional jabs at my already bruised and beaten ego. When someone says, "You look different," or "Damn, you're thin," I try not to let it get to me. But they're right—I've lost at least twenty pounds while I've been sick, a significant amount for someone who didn't have a lot of weight to lose. Though at five foot eight, one hundred and forty pounds, my body weight is relatively fine. I just have to force-feed myself while the nausea makes me want to vomit.

It's a frustrating situation that I try to hide from everyone, but it still makes me angry to realize that, while most people don't know I'm sick, they do know I've lost my muscular physique.

Tell them to fuck off. They don't care that you've spent countless hours in the gym sculpting a body you were proud of, and now, after less than a year of being sick, it's gone. They don't care that bodybuilding was your art form, that your masterpiece of a physique is ruined—a work-in-progress now working in reverse, deteriorating, muscle wasting away with each sedentary day. And they don't care how you feel about it. Shit, they don't care how you feel at all; they only care to point out that you don't look as good as you used to.

CHAPTER 20

This Is Depression

November 27, 2011

I've had this stupid illness for an entire year—more than half a million minutes. It's hard to remain hopeful when I haven't recovered yet, and it feels like I still have a long way to go. I need to take three more classes before I graduate, start teaching boot camp again, and get back to bodybuilding. But I'm afraid, legitimately scared, that none of that will happen. I fear this illness will never end, that it will be permanent, and I'll have to live the rest of my life missing out on the things I set out to do when I was healthy.

Part of this fear is rooted in my distrust in fate and what the future will hold. This illness has, in many ways, weakened my faith in the natural progression of my life and my ability to control my destiny. Perhaps that's why my mind is consumed by the possibility that there's nothing I can do to get better. I can't even find a doctor who knows how to treat chronic fatigue syndrome.

Even just thinking about living with this illness for another day makes me depressed, as if I'm trapped in a thick fog of discontentment. It's an unfamiliar and uncomfortable feeling, one of defeat. Depression, at least this level of it, is new to me. It makes me question when Dr. Gretchen blamed my illness on depression. My mental state back then was much happier, much more hopeful than it is today. Despite the trauma from the accident, I was still fairly upbeat, loving the life I had carved out for myself. That wasn't depression. *This* is depression. This toxic, weighty cloud hovering over me is the real depression. I'm trying to shake it off, or at least distract myself from it. Hopefully getting outside and taking a short bike ride will help lift the fog and change my mood.

In the driveway, I carefully straddle the Univega. But instead of sprinting down Mary Place, as I used to do, my cadence is slower. I coast past the tennis courts on Middlebrook and continue on, pedaling and thinking about my circumstances. I eventually ride up to the gym on campus, and my depression gets worse. I can barely stand looking at the wood awning, the big shiny windows, the racks of weights inside. It makes me sad and nostalgic to remember the countless hours I spent working out in that place. Now I have no strength, no energy to work out, and it makes me miss it even more. I miss everything about the gym—the sound of weights clanging together, the people bustling around, even the smell of sweat in the air. I miss losing myself in a world that few people can tolerate and even fewer people enjoy. It makes me remember staring out those big windows, looking at all the people outside hurrying around campus, occasionally making eye contact with them and wondering what they saw looking in. Now I know. I'm one of those people looking in, and I see my old self lost in a blissful world that once was mine. I owned that world, and with a passion so intense I would have let it kill me. Some days I wish it had.

I try not to let my emotions consume me as I ride on and make it to the north end of campus, where there's a deserted lot perfect for being depressed. Or just watching sunsets and thinking in solitude. The lot is close to where a new state-of-the-art concert hall is under construction. One day, probably soon, this abandoned lot likely will be developed also, but for now it remains my secret spot.

The sun is setting, but the pain in my legs from pedaling isn't. It continues to burn deep in my thighs and hamstrings while I sit on a discarded log among the weeds covering the empty lot. Still despondent about the struggles in my life, I take a deep breath, but it doesn't help. My chest feels heavy, as if I'm lying down while someone stands on top of me, as if my heart is breaking into a million little pieces and deteriorating into a fine dust, scattering all over the vacant lot.

I take out my phone and stare at it listlessly for a minute, then call my mom.

"Hey, sweetie . . ."

"Mom, I'm having bad thoughts. I've never felt like this, so hopeless. I guess I'm depressed."

"It's okay to be depressed," my mom says. "Depression is something a lot of people go through."

"I know, but the doctors blamed my illness on depression when I wasn't even that depressed. Now that I'm actually depressed, I feel like I can't acknowledge it, or the next doctor I see will do the same thing and just blame my symptoms on depression."

"I've seen your illness, and depression looks different," she says. "But maybe you have both; maybe you have a physical illness and depression. Being sick might even be making you depressed. That happens a lot, you know. Having an illness could make anyone depressed, even a happy person like you. And I think a good doctor will be able to see that."

"I hope so," I say, holding the phone up to my mouth.

"Do you want to tell me about your bad thoughts?" my mom asks.

"It just feels like I'm trying to buy time until I get better, but I'm not getting better."

"You *will* get better though. And you *are* getting better," she says. "It may be slow, but you are improving. Six months ago you couldn't have gone to school or even taken care of yourself. Now you're doing both of those things. That's progress."

"Yeah, I guess so," I say.

"And you know the depression won't last," my mom says. "Whatever you're feeling will eventually pass."

"I hope you're right."

"I am right." She chuckles into the phone. I laugh. It feels good to laugh.

After we hang up, I sit in the empty lot for half an hour, watching the last tinges of yellow, orange, and red fall below the horizon. The funk I've been in starts to fade, but my body is still recovering from the bike ride. I'm not sure if I have enough energy or strength to get home. Out of caution, I pedal slowly, using the lowest gear and coasting whenever possible.

On my way home, I pass a thicket of blackberry bushes lining a small creek, another hidden spot on campus that eventually leads to a bridge built of steel beams and wood planks. The planks shake the Univega's frame and rattle my legs as I continue to pedal. Then my tires find pavement and a small lake appears on the right. The water is serene, unfazed by its surroundings, completely at peace with everything under its surface. I continue riding through campus, but the thought of the lake stays with me. If only I could be at peace with my surroundings and everything under my surface.

YEAR 2

Renewed Experiences

CHAPTER 21

A Good Day

December 4, 2011

My illness has presented many challenges, but managing the sex drive of a twentysomething with no energy to spare is one of the most difficult. It feels as if, at any given time, I'm either too sick or too horny for my own good. Going almost a year without sex, or even so much as a kiss, has made my urges that much more intense. It's to be expected, but the urges still seem unusually intense and persistent for a sick person.

It could be a myth, but I've always thought that sick people naturally lose their sex drive. It seems like mine has only intensified, as if my brain is searching for a good feeling—something to mask the horrible feeling inside my body. With drugs, alcohol, and exercise proving too detrimental to my illness, sometimes an orgasm is the only pleasure I can handle. Even so, satisfying the urge is not without consequence—my attempts at self-pleasure are riddled by false starts and post-orgasm malaise. Even the smallest amount of sexual stimulation can put my body in a tailspin. There is, however, a brief moment when it feels the way it should, like standing atop a mountain or cashing a big paycheck, but with more euphoria, much like, well, having actual sex—healthy person sex. But when the feeling fades, a painful, burning sensation fills my muscles and joints. Then the weakness takes over, rendering my body useless and full of a rotten feeling pinned so deep in my stomach it seems like it could actually burn through my spine. It's enough to make me swear off all future sexual urges. That is, until out of boredom, I search online for photos of Scarlett Johansson and my body flares with symptoms again. Because of this, I've started setting the parental controls on my laptop and smartphone. This way there's no porn to look at, or even a sexy photo that might trigger my urges and the physical consequences that follow them.

The adverse reaction I get to sexual stimulation makes me feel timid about starting a relationship with anyone, especially a sexual one. I don't know how my body will react in such a situation. When I'm alone I can deal with it, but I don't want to scare my partner with a tremor attack, like the one I had with Molly. She has since moved on to a new boyfriend. I too must move on, which means I will eventually need to decide whether to try to have sex again, a dilemma that I may face sooner than I would like.

I've been chatting online with Sasha, who also goes to Sonoma State. Despite knowing many of the same people, we've never met. We do have a lot in common though—an unabashed fondness for romantic comedies and sappy love songs, a mild obsession for eating healthy, and an intense passion for fitness. I just hope that the conversations we've had online will translate to equally good chemistry when we meet in person for the first time later today.

After sitting on the couch for an hour, pretending to do homework on my porn-free computer, I drive to a local coffee shop to meet Sasha. I'm not sure if it's a date, so I arrive early and place my order without her. I want it to be a date, but I'm afraid of the awkwardness—should I offer to pay for her? And if so, how do I offer without drawing attention from everyone around us?

Even more than the awkwardness, I'm afraid of letting Sasha into my life. I haven't told her that I'm sick, and I'd like to avoid doing so, ideally forever. Having the "I'm not the healthiest guy in the world" conversation is something I've been dreading. But if I don't tell her and we get intimate, she'll be completely blindsided, maybe even traumatized—though it's unlikely that the date will get that far. Sasha already seemed annoyed with me during our last conversation, probably because I've been putting off meeting her, stalling because I didn't want to make plans and be too sick to show up.

As I'm sitting in the coffee shop waiting for Sasha, I hear my name called out from the register. On the counter, I find a cup of tea and a receipt with "Jameson" written on it. I grab my order and turn to see Sasha standing in front of me.

"Hiya, whatcha got there?" she asks, looking down at my tea.

"Oh, hi. It's herbal tea."

"Looks good. I'm gonna get one," Sasha says. "I'll come find you."

"Great, I'm over there." I point to the table I was sitting at in a corner of the coffee shop, then walk toward it.

Sasha orders while I sit with my tea and awkwardly stare at her. She looks lovely—her hair, brown with blond highlights, her big doe eyes, her sweet smile accented by a dime-sized dimple on her left cheek.

She walks over and sits down at the table with her tea. "Hi. How's the tea?"

"It's good," I say. "Did you try yours?"

"Yeah, I like it."

There's a long silence as we both drink from our cups, but Sasha's soft yet spirited voice remains in my head. And it's not just her voice that I like; there's something about her demeanor that makes me feel attractive and wanted, even kind of sexy. It's how I felt on my first date with Molly, and how I used to feel posing on stage during a bodybuilding competition or in front of a photographer's camera. I've missed this feeling.

"So, what have you been up to?" I take a sip of tea and look over at her.

"I just finished cheer practice," she says.

"Oh, cool. You coach the cheer team, right? How's that going?"

"Good. But it's weird being a coach. I'm used to being on the team." Sasha shrugs, then looks at me curiously. "How 'bout you? What have you been doing?"

"Not much," I say. "Just finishing the semester."

"How many classes are you taking?" Sasha asks.

"I'm just taking one," I confess.

"Oh, is it your last class? Are you graduating this semester?"

"Um, no. I still need three more classes to graduate."

"Then why are you only taking one class?" she asks.

I'm worried that no good will come from the truth. If I tell her I'm sick, she'll either pity me and I'll lose my attractiveness, or she'll think I'm faking my illness. My instinct is to make up an excuse, like I'm trying to extend my stay at Sonoma State by only taking one class at a time, but that sounds idiotic, and I'm a horrible liar. It's a no-win situation, so I should at least be honest.

"I got mono last year," I say. "So I'm taking it easy this semester."

"Oh, that sucks," she says. "But good for you for knowing your limits. How are you feeling now?"

"I have good days and bad days." I glance down at my tea and take a sip.

"Is today a good day?" Sasha asks.

I look up from my tea. "Well, I'm here with you, not home in bed. So yeah, today is a good day."

CHAPTER 22

Bottleneck

December 5, 2011

After opening my eyes, I roll over to an empty space in my bed. I had a good time with Sasha yesterday, but it was for the best that our date ended at the coffee shop. My body wasn't ready for anything sexual, and it was a relief that nothing else happened between us. Not to mention, I didn't have time for it. I had work to do on the group presentation, which is scheduled for later today.

Last night I met with my group at the Sonoma State library. I was exhausted from the date with Sasha and couldn't drive myself, but luckily Thomas was around to give me a ride. Walking from the parking lot to Charlie Brown's Café and up the stairs to the second floor of the library was enough to do me in, but I still needed to finish my part of the presentation and didn't want to look like a slacker for not showing up. So I stubbornly pressed on, and after trudging past several rows of computers, I finally found the other group members in the back of the building.

The bright lights and raised thermostat in the library made concentrating on my work feel like reading a book with my feet in a broiler and halogen lights in my eyes. I was lucky to make it an hour in that place. And Shelly, the unofficial leader of the group, didn't make it any easier. She acted like a real fascist.

She ordered everyone around as if she were teaching the class and gave me suspicious looks anytime I took a break. Normally I would have given her an earful of witty comebacks and sarcastic retorts, but I didn't want to waste my energy. So I just sat next to the other people in the group and let Shelly obsess over giving orders. It was necessary for me to keep my distance from her and the repercussions of her delegating, which is why I remained seated almost the entire time and yielded as many tasks as I could to more able-bodied members of the group without being obvious or obnoxious.

While Shelly spouted off orders, I joined the other two group members' universal boycott of her forced leadership. Though she still managed to spur our attention with choleric questions like, "Do you understand what I'm saying?" and "Can you handle that?" I'm not sure which one of us she was talking to, but I don't think it mattered to her, or us—we were one collective blob of subordination. In fairness, her questions weren't always condescending. Well, actually, they probably were; I just wasn't paying enough attention to tell for sure. Listening and talking to Shelly took a level of patience and energy that I didn't have. Like the others in the group, when she looked at me, I just nodded and mumbled an affirmation reprised from my adolescence—*umm-uh-huh*.

Now, fourteen hours later, after a wakeful sleep, I'm struggling to recover from all the activity. If I can just get through the presentation this afternoon without my health taking a dive, there will be a passing grade for me, and I will have accomplished a major milestone on my journey back to health.

As a precaution, so I don't jeopardize my ability to do the presentation, I sit on the carpet near the sliding glass door in the living room and rest. But trying to rest feels impossible when my nerves are so taut. Waiting for the presentation makes me nervous, too nervous to distract myself with TV or video games, so I lie on the floor with my head resting on a foam roller and try to catch glimpses of the tennis matches across the street. It's energy conservation at its most challenging or most pathetic—one of the two, maybe both.

When hunger hits, I snack on a bowl of granola, hoping it's enough sustenance to get me through two hours of class. Then I take out some notecards and read over my part of the presentation. I have the words memorized but I need something to focus on so I stop worrying about whether my body will hold up for the next few hours.

My phone says it's almost noon, and the presentation is at one. The next half hour goes by so slowly it almost feels as if time is being added to the clock, and checking my phone every two minutes doesn't help. Finally I grab my backpack, mount the Univega, and ride down Mary Place, pedaling sparingly and coasting whenever possible—*pedal, coast, coast, coast, pedal, coast, coast, coast.*

At the main entrance to campus, there's a shortcut through Sauvignon, one of Sonoma State's student dorms named after viticultural terms. Freshmen year I lived in Verdot, a dorm on the shabbier side, at least compared to the radiant heat flooring, full kitchens, and granite countertops of Beaujolais and the newly built Tuscany.

While pedaling through Sauvignon, my head gets dizzy, my lungs begin to wheeze, and my muscles burn. This is how it's supposed to feel running up a steep hill with ankle weights on, not slowly riding my bike a few blocks.

About a hundred yards up ahead, there's a crosswalk leading to the center of campus. On the right, I see a man riding his bike, approaching the crosswalk perpendicularly. He's pedaling fast, much faster than me. It looks like we're going to enter the crosswalk at the same time, but I don't have the strength to speed up, and I'm already going as slowly as I can without stopping.

We try not to crash, or at least I try not to, as the other guy seems intent on remaining oblivious to a potential collision. I'm about to run right into him, but at the last second, I swerve and wobble my bike alongside his. He's still ignoring me, and, for about fifty-feet, we continue to pedal side-by-side while I struggle to straighten my steering. Then I hit a pothole and fall off my bike onto a patch of dirt on the sidewalk. It's not an epic crash, not like the time I rode the Univega drunk through a darkened parking lot full of speed bumps, but it's a crash nonetheless, and one that is certainly memorable for its awkwardness and horrible timing.

Once I pick myself up and brush the dirt off my jeans, I grab the Univega and prop it against a nearby tree. Then I sit at the base of the tree and take out my phone to check the time. It's nearly one o'clock. My class is about to start, and I'm out of breath, too shaken up and in too much pain to ride my bike.

I warily walk the rest of the way to class, pushing the Univega and shaking my head the whole way. After locking the bike to a light pole in front of a large two-story building, I hobble upstairs to a crowded room at the end of a long hallway and sit down surrounded by a cacophony of loud voices. I take a few breaths, trying to focus on just sitting here in class and what an accomplishment it is—how getting this far was physically impossible a year ago. But before I feel too accomplished, the other members of my group walk toward the front of the class, and I lift my throbbing body out of my chair and follow them.

We are presenting on the leadership styles demonstrated in the movie *Saving Private Ryan*. Our presentation is accompanied by PowerPoint slides, which need to be operated by someone in the group sitting at the class computer. The job comes with a big comfy chair to sit in. I want that job. No, I need that job. But because I'm too proud, or too slow, someone else gets to it before me. I settle for leaning against the wall to take some of the weight off my muscles. It's easier than standing upright, but it's not the most professional posture.

Shelly sees me on the wall and gives me a disapproving look. "Jamison, come stand over here, away from the wall," she says, like a schoolteacher scolding her student.

"I'm good right here," I say, my voice soft so I don't attract attention from anyone else. I give Shelly a look of contempt though, and she scowls at me.

Oh, she did not like that. She's pissed.

The tension between us is palpable. Shelly's glare projects onto me like the summer sun on a black car. While she may not like to be defied, there's no way I'm going to let her demands impede my one shot at passing this course. And I'm definitely not going to further jeopardize my health by giving in to her demands. Neither she nor anyone else in the class know I'm sick. A few weeks ago, I did try to tell the professor about my illness, but she was in a hurry and barely acknowledged what I told her. She, and my classmates, probably think I'm just being lazy or trying to look cool by leaning against the wall. They don't realize that this is necessary for me. It's not a choice. It's survival—I'm just trying to stay on my feet long enough to pull off a passing grade, long enough to show that my health has improved, and I can get on with my life.

You don't have to power through this. Go ahead, lean against the wall. Fuck, sit on the damn floor if it gets you through the presentation. The alternative is much worse. If you get sicker—you know, like when you start seeing funny shapes and feel like you're going to pass out—everyone will just think you want attention. You'll collapse in front of the whole class, and they'll think you're trying to get the professor to excuse you from the assignment. Nobody will know that you are legitimately sick.

After ten minutes of standing awkwardly against the wall like a lonely freshman at the Homecoming dance, I step forward and all eyes in the room focus on me, all eyes that are still awake, that is. Clutching my crumpled note cards, I glance back to the projection screen. Everything seems to be in order, everything except my body. A sharp tremor shoots across my torso. *Shit.* Another one jolts my legs.

I start to speak and realize that the tremors are jarring me so hard that my teeth are chattering and the keys in my pants are jingling. It sounds like I'm trying to give a speech while standing barefoot on a frozen lake with little bells attached to my feet. With a few slow breaths, the tremors gradually settle down and my teeth stop chattering. For several seconds, the room is eerily quiet. I should probably finish what I was saying, but I don't want the tremors to start again.

Looking down at my note cards, I slowly start to speak again. Words are coming out of my mouth—something about Tom Hanks's character and authoritative leadership. Hopefully what I'm saying makes sense; hopefully I sound coherent. I don't feel coherent. I feel sick and disoriented, impaired by the illness. There's a bottleneck somewhere in my body, and my brain is trying to allocate the necessary resources, mostly blood, to keep my body upright and somewhat functional so I can finish my part of the presentation. Thankfully, it's almost over. Just a few more minutes and I'll be done.

After ending with a cheesy joke, I'm cued to return to my seat by the professor's praise and claps from my now awoken but still half-conscious classmates. My stride walking from the front of the class feels limp and achy—one leg is limp, the other is achy.

When the professor ends class, I lean back in my chair, my eyes closed, a smile on my face. The tremors start up again, but I don't care. They can shake me all they want, for I've accomplished what I came here to do—I've finished the semester, and now I'm one step closer to graduating. I want to celebrate at a bar with Thomas and James or throw a party at our house, but that would surely make me feel worse, probably as sick as I was after last year's Christmas party.

As a consolation, I reach into my backpack, pull out a can of coconut water, and pretend it's a cold, hoppy beer. It's not the same, not at all, but it's still refreshing, with little chunks of coconut meat floating around the milky fluid. I savor it until the last sip. Then, finally, I'm ready to go home.

Now all you have to do is not crash your bike.

CHAPTER 23

A Different Bridge

January 20, 2012

Today I'm moving for the fifth time in five years, this time to my mom's house in Tuolumne. I've been dreading it for weeks, and not just because I'm going to miss living on my own. Moving is a pain in the ass. It started last week with packing—individually wrapping each item in newspaper, placing it carefully in a box, then repeating that a few dozen times before neatly organizing all the boxes in a corner of my room, and finally carrying the damn things out of what used to be my perfectly nested dwelling.

Before packing and moving my stuff, I got rid of many items, mostly large furniture and exercise equipment. It was fascinating to see the types of people who responded to the ads I put on Craigslist. There was the older woman who got a little pushy when she realized I was giving away a bed frame without a mattress. There was the middle-aged, musky gentleman with dreadlocks who needed a shower. He packed my sofa chair into an unmarked, marijuana-scented van with a disoriented dog in the back. When the man opened the van's sliding door, the dog bolted out and started running up and down the street as if she were on a bad acid trip, or more likely, a weed high. Then there were the two beer-bellied drinking buddies, who exuberantly snatched up my exceedingly heavy, decade-old TV—an ancestor of the slimmer models now on the market. Finally, just a few minutes ago, there was the Petaluma family who hauled off my beloved tractor tire—yes, beloved.

How much love can someone have for a three-hundred-pound mass of conglomerated rubber? A lot—certainly as much as, if not more than, the obsession a child has for an action figure or dollhouse. The tractor tire was my instrument of hobby, my fitness plaything. For hours—many hours—I would flip it end over end on the backyard patio, creating a reverberating *slap*, then another *slap*. The sound would bounce off the siding of the house and make a sort of instrumental warrior cry, which was often answered by the sound of tennis balls being batted around across the street. The neighbors must have been thrilled listening to the sounds: *slap, slap, whack, whack, slap, slap, whack, whack.*

When the family arrived to take the tire away, I helped them lift it into their truck—a bad idea for a sick person with a whole day of carrying heavy things ahead of him. Before leaving, the father told me he had been working on a backyard playground for his son. It had taken him nearly a year, and the tractor tire was the final addition. The sentiment made me feel better about parting with something that had been so integral to my own backyard fun.

Now I sit and recover on the curb in front of the house, waiting for my dad to arrive with his truck, so we can load up my stuff. In his late-fifties, my dad resembles a relative of Santa

Claus and Jerry Garcia, with a thick gray beard and his hair tied back in a ponytail.

I've always had a loving relationship with my dad, but we're not as close as we were when I was younger. He and my mom separated when I was an infant, so I spent most of my childhood switching off between their houses. When I stayed with my dad, all our free time revolved around sports. Almost every day we'd find a baseball diamond and he'd hit me ground balls and pop flies until I was delirious. My dad would stand at home plate with a backward baseball cap and his shirt off, a gnarly scar running down his abdomen from the cancer he had removed a few years earlier. Then he'd hit me a ball at shortstop and I'd throw it back to him, making sure to keep track of how many balls I had fielded consecutively.

Back then we spent countless hours watching baseball games and collecting sports cards, but when I grew older and went to high school and college, it became harder for us to stay close. He's been there when I've needed him, like when he drove up to see me after the car accident, and I still regularly talk to him on the phone, but now we only see each other a few times a year.

When my dad pulls up in front of my house, he starts to load boxes in the back of his truck. I'm still exhausted from moving the tractor tire, so my contribution consists of bringing a box out to the truck, then walking back inside and resting for fifteen minutes before doing it again. While I'm recovering, Thomas and my dad move my boxes, small furnishings, and a mattress, all before I'm able to make two trips to the truck. It makes me feel weak and inferior. I hate it.

As I continue to rest on the couch, I try to figure out how I'm going to get through the rest of the day. I need to summon the strength to clean my room, drive four hours to my mom's house, and then unload my stuff later this evening. Thankfully

Thomas wants to help. He's going to drive the Xterra to Tuolumne, help unload my stuff, then travel back to Sonoma tomorrow with my dad to clean the house, all for a free dinner and a few bucks. He's a good friend, my best friend.

I'm going to miss living with Thomas—walking to the park and throwing his frisbee around, or grabbing our baseball gloves and playing catch in the street while trying not to hit any parked cars. I'm going to miss coming home and seeing Thomas sitting in front of the TV, binge-watching *How I Met Your Mother*. I'm even going to miss nagging him about doing his dishes. I'm going to miss it all, but I know it's time to move on, time to leave our lives in Sonoma behind.

We watch the garage door rattle to the ground one last time, and my mind is full of suppressed emotions and clichéd thoughts. But I also get a feeling of discontent for how unsettled my life is, how uncertain everything feels. It's hard to leave Sonoma like this without a guarantee that I'll finish my degree or stay connected to my friends. And then there's Sasha. While we still talk almost every day, we haven't had a second date yet. I'm nervous and a bit cynical about our courtship. I don't know if she understands how sick I am and what her life would look like attached to mine. We plan to have lunch again soon, but it's frustrating to leave now and create such distance between us—she'll be in Sonoma, a four-hour drive from my mom's house in Tuolumne.

As for getting my diploma, I'll take my remaining classes online. I'd prefer to take them on campus, but I can't afford to keep inching along like I did this semester. Even so, leaving now feels premature, like putting down a book mid-page.

You'll be done in a couple months, after you take the online classes. All that matters is you finished this semester. It may not feel like it, but you're done with college. This is your graduation, the culmination of your life so far—the dedication, the struggles, the achievements, the grueling days before you got sick, the even more grueling days after you got sick. Everything has led to this moment.

We drive down Mary Place and along my familiar bike route on Middlebrook and Bodway. I'm overcome with sadness as I leave Sonoma State, the place that has been my home for the last five years. My entire adult life has been rooted here. This is where I started bodybuilding, where I got my fitness instructor certification, and where I dealt with the aftermath of the car accident. I completed so many rites of passage here. Now, as I drive away, it's hard to leave it all behind.

* * *

As Thomas and I drive along the bay, he plays his favorite Christian rock band on the car stereo. Wind is rippling over the water as it shimmers with an almost metallic gloss. My window is partway down, letting a rush of cold air whip through the car as we drive onto the Richmond Bridge, its steel beams towering above us. I look at the side of the bridge, the metal railing whizzing by and the water drifting below. Suddenly I'm confronted by the familiar but terrifying feeling of being on a different bridge—the Napa River Bridge—humming along to my favorite tunes, blissfully unaware of the tragedy on the horizon. Then it hits me, or rather I hit it—fate, destruction, death.

Something in the passenger's side-view mirror snaps me out of the trance. My dad is driving directly behind us, and a rectangular object is sticking straight up from the bed of his truck. Whatever the object, it must be seven or eight feet tall, and it's being forced into a vertical position by the draft coming off the bridge. The object looks like it's about to fly away, and it's held down only by a frayed rope that's sure to snap and send it darting into traffic like a giant throwing star. Something violent and catastrophic is about to happen—there will be blood and broken glass everywhere, property will be damaged, lives will be ended, and my dad will be in the middle of it all. I don't think I could handle losing him right now.

Take a deep breath, think logically—act, don't react. You could be imagining this, or it could be real, like the time you were driving with Keith and Tony and the guy ran over the streetlamp while having a heart attack. It's a little odd that Thomas hasn't noticed anything. Ask him to look at the truck and see what he says. It can't hurt. The worst case is that he has no idea what you're talking about, and you feel a little crazy.

I turn to Thomas and nudge his arm with my elbow.

"Hey, hey man, look in the rearview . . ." I nod upward.

"Yeah, okay . . . what is that?" he asks.

I turn around in my seat to get a better look. "I don't know. I can't tell."

"Wait, man, is that the mattress?" Thomas asks, as a racket of car horns blares behind us.

"Let me call my dad." I swipe at my phone's screen and tap my dad's number. He picks up. "Dad, is my mattress about to fly off the truck?"

"Yeah, I need to get to the other side of the bridge. There's nowhere to pull over," he says, distracted by car horns. "I can't concentrate with all these fucking people honking at me. I gotta go, son."

We pull over at the first turnoff on the Richmond side of the bridge. My dad parks behind us, and the queen-sized mattress slams down on the bed of the truck. He gets out and ties it down, using a few extra precautions this time. Then Thomas walks over to talk to him while I stay in the car, saving my strength to unload boxes later. I look at the driver's seat and flip down the overhead visor. The hospital bracelet is still there, still serving its purpose. I hold the bracelet for a few seconds before Thomas walks back toward the car and I quickly reattach it to the visor.

"Wow, that could have been really bad," Thomas says, getting back in the Xterra.

"I know, right? How did it not fly away?" I say.

"Must have been the music we were listening to," Thomas says with a smile on his face. He continues playing his Christian rock as we drive off, making our way past the bridge's toll plaza en route to Tuolumne.

CHAPTER 24

The Doctor I've Been Looking For

May 11, 2012

After finishing my remaining courses online, I'm officially done with college. My advisor at Sonoma State said I should receive my diploma by the end of the year. Now I have to transition into the workforce. But because I'm still sick, there's no office job, or any other on-site employment, that I'm capable of doing. Though, I have found some work as a freelance writer composing articles, blog posts, and other types of web content. The articles are mainly for company websites, and they're pretty boring, but occasionally there's an intriguing topic to write about with a headline like, "The Best Portable Toilets in New York."

I have to tailor my work schedule to how my body feels, which usually means working about twenty-five hours a week. The pay is lousy, around three cents for every word I write, but I can work at my own pace, any time of the day, from anywhere that has an internet connection.

In addition to writing web content, I've been using my time to process some of the residual trauma from the car accident, which for the last year and a half has been largely overshadowed by the stress of my illness. In many ways, being sick has interrupted my healing process and consumed my life in a way that has made it hard to even think about the accident. But now that my health is a bit better, I'm finally getting back to healing the emotional wounds.

I've been talking to my mom about the guilt I feel from the accident. I don't blame myself for everything that happened, but it's hard not to feel at least partially responsible when someone's life was lost. I just wish I had done something to avoid crashing on the bridge that day. But as my mom has pointed out, if I had avoided crashing, someone else might not have been as lucky and could have died along with the other driver. When I think about it like that, I'm glad it was my car that crashed and not one full of people.

It's insights like these that make me recognize the importance of talking about the accident. Opening up about it has given me new perspectives that I never would have realized had I kept my thoughts and feelings bottled up. Seeing a new therapist has also helped me open up. Ellen, a middle-aged woman with a kind face and graying, dark, frizzy hair, is much more helpful than the psychiatrist I saw a couple years ago, the guy I paid one hundred dollars an hour to talk about sports.

Every Wednesday for the last three months, my mom has dropped me off at Ellen's office in Sonora, a small town near Tuolumne, and we've talked for an hour about whatever has been on my mind. I've sat on her long blue couch, with her across from me in a creaky old rocker, and I've purged my feelings about the car accident and the struggles I've had with my illness.

One of the first things I asked Ellen was if I have post-traumatic stress disorder. She told me that I probably do, but suggested I not focus on the label because PTSD is an umbrella term used for many kinds of trauma. She said that it would be better for me to focus on my individual case, rather than compare it to a broad swath of other cases.

During one session, Ellen asked me if I ever think about the man who died in the accident. I told her that sometimes I do, but because I never knew him, it's usually out of curiosity. I don't know where he grew up, what his family was like, or how he spent his free time. I don't even know what he looked like. I saw his name a few times on the accident report and insurance forms, but I've since forgotten it. I think he was relatively young, in his late-thirties, but that's all I know about the person I killed. And it's why, when I do think about him, my thoughts are filled with questions—who was he and why was his car stopped in the middle of the highway?

Ellen told me that I may never know why he stopped on the bridge that day. But that's okay. She showed me that I don't need to pressure myself to find that kind of closure. She said that unanswered questions often go along with traumatic events like car accidents, but as time goes on, it'll get easier to cope with the unknown.

It was therapeutic, even cathartic, to hear her say that, because I've felt so much pressure from myself and other people to recover from the trauma of the accident. It feels good to know that I don't have to reach some mythical end to my coping. Just like any other bad memory, the accident is something that will stay with me for the rest of my life, but acknowledging that is better than any closure I could search for and force myself to find.

With Ellen's help, I've made significant progress in coping with the car accident. I have fewer flashbacks now, and reminders of the accident don't bother me as much. The other night, I watched *Zodiac*, starring Jake Gyllenhaal, and right there in the opening scene was an aerial shot of the Napa River Bridge. It surprised me that a random bridge in Northern California was in a major Hollywood movie, but even more surprising was the fact that it didn't trigger any traumatic episodes or horrifying nightmares. I told Ellen about it, and she said it was inevitable that I'd notice something like that, but it was a good sign that I didn't have an intense emotional reaction. "That's progress," she told me.

I've really enjoyed my sessions with Ellen, but now, unfortunately, she's moving her practice to a bigger city, and I won't be able to see her anymore. That's okay, though. I'm glad I've had a chance to work with her. During our final session together, she recommended a few books for me to read, like *Half a Life*, a memoir by Darin Strauss, who was in a similar car accident. She also urged me to research chronic fatigue syndrome, the illness Dr. Gretchen diagnosed me with, and look for a medical doctor who can treat it.

I started my search by reading through online articles and forums about the illness, many of which mentioned something called myalgic encephalomyelitis, a neurological disease that is the same as, or similar to, chronic fatigue syndrome. Some of the articles focused on a theory that the Epstein-Barr virus, which causes mononucleosis, is also at the root of CFS. The idea is that the virus attacks the body's mitochondria, leeching the cellular energy they produce and thus making a person sick with CFS. This mitochondrial dysfunction would explain why I've been so weak and fatigued for such a long time. It might also explain some of my other symptoms, like the body tremors.

In my online research, I was unable to find any helpful treatments. I did, however, find a kinship with other people who have been diagnosed with chronic fatigue syndrome, or myalgic encephalomyelitis, or whatever the hell my illness is called. One forum post from someone named Lizzie in the United Kingdom gave me hope. She wrote about finding peace in the inevitable difficulties of the illness, and joy in simple things like wearing shoes after being bedridden for a week or how the sunshine feels on her face when she goes outside. I've read her post at least three times today. It's my way of ignoring the sad stories of people with this illness who have been sick for years, some even decades. The thought of being sick that long, with any illness, is frightening.

I've been sick for a year and a half, a fraction of what many people with CFS go through, and yet the illness has already done so much damage to my life. I can only imagine what sort of destruction it could cause after ten or twenty years. This is the reality of people living with CFS and other chronic illnesses, many of whom have lost faith in their doctors, and the medical establishment as a whole, because their conditions haven't improved.

As someone who has thrived on fitness and a healthy lifestyle, I never thought I would one day have to live with a chronic illness. But that's the case for many people with mysterious health conditions. Some people may be born with chronic illnesses, others may acquire them later in life, but we all must live with a devastating condition for which doctors have few answers, if any.

I've always relied on the idea that modern medicine would be able to treat, or at least identify, any illness that I acquire in my lifetime. Now I'm a bit more disenchanted, but I will not give up hope. I refuse to believe that there's nobody, no researcher or medical doctor, who understands my illness. That's why, with some encouragement from Ellen, I've restarted my search to find a CFS specialist.

And I may have just found the doctor I've been looking for. Dr. Daniel Peterson in Lake Tahoe is one of the leading clinicians seeing CFS patients. His name is mentioned in *The New York Times*, best-selling books, and *I Remember Me*, a documentary that profiles some of the history of the illness. Dr. Peterson's ardent work has shed some light on potential treatments for CFS, and many patients think he's brilliant, so I'm going to give him a shot.

As soon as I find the number to his office, I make the call.

"Hello?" a soft male voice says on the other end of the phone.

"Hi, I would like to make an appointment with Dr. Peterson."

"Sure, are you a regular patient, or do you have CFS?"

"I have CFS, but I've never seen Dr. Peterson."

"Okay, first you need a referral from your general practitioner," the man says. I hear papers shuffling around in the background. "In the meantime, I'll send you paperwork to fill out. It will cover what to expect during your first visit, your health history, the cost of the appointment, you know, stuff like that. So fill out the paperwork, send it back to us with the referral, then we'll get you set up with an appointment."

Filling out paperwork and going to see another doctor before I drive four hours to see Dr. Peterson sounds exhausting. If I were healthy, the process wouldn't be that bad, but then again, if I were healthy, I wouldn't need to see a doctor at all. It's a frustrating paradox.

The receptionist emails me the paperwork, which I fill out and send back to him. Then I make an appointment to get a referral from a local doctor and hope the rest of the process goes smoothly. I'm ready for Dr. Peterson to help me, so I can finally be done with this illness.

CHAPTER 25

Saliva Is Everywhere

June 25, 2012

The day starts with me and my mom getting lost in Incline Village, an affluent community on the shore of Lake Tahoe, where Dr. Peterson has his medical practice. I call the doctor's receptionist, and he explains that we've driven to the doctor's former office—a musty, deserted building that smells like cigarettes and moldy carpet. It looks like a prison for has-been lawyers.

The receptionist tells us how to get to the new office, and we arrive at a much cleaner and more modern building. The lobby has a sleek reception desk, high ceilings, and a door leading to a patio shaded by tall trees. My mom and I sit in the waiting room for what seems like an hour, until a nurse ushers me away to take my vitals. Then we wait once again, this time in a small exam room. The clock on my phone says it's around noon, my appointment was supposed to start at eleven fifteen.

Finally, a man wearing a collared shirt and slacks enters the room. He's portly, clean shaven, and balding with sparse hairs combed over his shiny scalp. The man doesn't say anything except, "Good morning," then sits down and digs into a file full of papers.

It takes this unfamiliar man sitting in front of me to realize that I'm not entirely sure what Dr. Peterson looks like. The images I saw of him online were at least two decades old. He was young, thin, and had a neatly trimmed mustache and a full head of brown hair. The man who just walked in the room looks nothing like that. Assuming the man is indeed Dr. Peterson, he's either incredibly distracted, or of the assumption that I already know what he looks like, as if his face is instantly recognizable, even to a new patient.

After a couple minutes of extremely awkward silence, and as if making an entirely separate entrance, the man says, "I'm Dr. Peterson." Another long pause settles in the room before he finally asks, "Do you remember your initial episode of mono?"

"I do—it started in the middle of a workout, just totally blindsided me. I started getting really sick. I felt dizzy, like I was going to pass out. But I didn't stop the workout; I kept going. Then I had heart palpitations, and that night I had chills and cold sweats."

"That was in December of 2010?" The doctor scribbles something in his notes.

"Yeah, it was right after Thanksgiving."

"And you've basically stayed sick since then?" Dr. Peterson asks.

"That's right," I say.

"You know, normally patients have to wait much longer to see me," the doctor says. "But one of the reasons I upped you on my waiting list is that, in the twenty-five years I've been doing this, I've learned that the longer you wait, the longer you stay sick. And if this was going to be a short-duration illness, you would have gotten well a long time ago. You'll see some other patients around here who have been sick fifteen or twenty years, and they started just like you. It's, you know, a bad story." Dr. Peterson pauses and looks at me confidently. "Here's what I've learned: The quicker you get the information and intervene, the better chances you have at a full recovery. And then this just looks like a couple years that you had a bad case of mono. Okay?"

"Okay," I say. "That makes sense." I'm inspired by the possibility of finally recovering from this illness and interested to hear Dr. Peterson's plan.

"I have learned to do whatever we can to aggressively intervene. I will measure exactly why you're fatigued, where it's coming from, and what you can do about it. If I were to wave my magic wand and make the fatigue go away, would you still have some residual things going on?"

"Yeah, but life would be a lot easier," I say.

"Did you ever think that you could exercise through this?" the doctor asks.

"I tried to. I feel like that might have made it worse."

"It *did* make it worse," he says. "It's a very common thing, especially for young men. They have—"

"A need to power through it," I say, finishing the doctor's thought.

"Yes, and they usually make themselves worse, sometimes for a prolonged period of time." The doctor pauses and looks around the room contemplatively. "Let me tell you what I know about this disease: not all cases are caused by the Epstein-Barr virus, although yours probably was. That's one thing I will figure out. Did you have any contact with people who had mono before you got sick?"

"My roommate James had it when he was younger, but I don't remember being exposed to anyone who had it at the time that I got sick."

"Any intimate contact?"

"Just with my girlfriend at the time." I don't know whether Molly had ever had mono, but, theoretically, I could have gotten it from her.

"And you were training at the gym, so you had contact with a lot of people there?"

"That's right."

"This illness is very difficult to trace, but we think it can be contagious to people who've never had it. So, someone could have given it to you, and you could pass it on to someone else in the future. It really depends on the contact you have with a person, and whether they were exposed to the illness in the past," Dr. Peterson explains.

"Oh, okay." I nod my head. Then Dr. Peterson stands up and asks my mom to step out of the room, leaving the two of us alone.

"Is there anything you want to tell me that you couldn't with her here?" the doctor asks.

I give him a confused look. "No, not that I can think of . . . Why?"

"Okay, great. It's just that sometimes people have concerns about sexual contact they had and not everyone feels comfortable talking about it in front of family members."

"Oh, gotcha. I was only intimate with my girlfriend. Well, now she's my ex-girlfriend. And I don't know if she ever had mono."

"Right, well, depending on the circumstances, your girlfriend at the time, or even just a fling you had a month before getting sick, could have given you the virus," the doctor says.

"The same goes if you were to now have a girlfriend—there's a chance you could give her the illness."

This is partly why I've been hesitant to be intimate with Sasha. I don't want to get her sick. "So how do I know if I'll give someone the illness?"

"It's difficult to know for sure, but if the person is susceptible, it can spread through kissing. Although in any individual case, it could also be some fluke. Saliva is transferred more easily than we think."

"I know. Saliva is everywhere." I think back to all the times in college when I kissed people at parties or shared drinks without giving it a second thought.

"The thing is, you were just as likely to have gotten mono by being spit on at the gym as you were from a sexual partner."

"That's a lovely image," I say. "But it's what I figured—I got it from sharing a drink or something."

"It could have been any number of ways," the doctor interjects. "As I said, saliva is how it's transmitted."

"Right."

Dr. Peterson walks over to me and gives me a quick physical exam, then welcomes my mom back into the room.

The doctor sits down and looks at me. "What I'm going to do today is measure your fatigue, and we do that by the standard protocol for fatigue measurement—VO$_2$ max. As a fitness trainer, you're probably familiar with this exercise test. I do it because I want you to be fatigued enough that I can find what's wrong, but I don't want to kill you."

"Good." I laugh. "I don't want you to kill me either."

"Don't worry, I'll be around to monitor you, and we'll see how you do," Dr. Peterson says. "And just so you know, this disease lives in your immune system. That's why it wasn't just a short illness. There's something different about your immune system. We're going to learn one of two things: it was either a concomitant event—you made yourself worse trying to exercise through it, but if you had just gone home and gone to bed for a few weeks you would have been fine—or you were genetically predisposed to the illness. I will measure that and tell you which one is the case. The results obviously have implications for the future."

"Right," I say politely.

"You would have had a spontaneous recovery by now if it were going to happen, and there's no exceptions to that, whether you believe the Dubbo studies or not," the doctor says. I nod, even though I have no idea what the Dubbo studies are. "The studies were sponsored by the CDC and the Australian government. They are pretty dense with data but show that about ten percent of the participants with mono still had debilitating symptoms after six months."

"Wow, that's me—I'm the ten percent."

"Yes," Dr. Peterson says. "Needless to say we must do something if you want to get better."

"When you say 'something,' what do you mean?" I look at the doctor.

"Immune modulation, antivirals, a combination of the two; Coenzyme Q10, gamma globulin, things like that."

"Okay, gotcha," I say, still pretending to know what he's talking about.

"All right, so, in a few minutes we will have you do the VO_2 max test."

"Is it running or biking?" I ask, trying to prove I actually know something.

"You get to choose, but for somebody like yourself, I would run. A bike, as you probably know, underestimates by about twelve percent. For an older, out of shape adult like myself, it really doesn't make a difference, but for you, I really want accurate data."

"Okay, I'm up for that."

"It's going to make you sick, but that's what I'm trying to do. Unfortunately, it's a necessary part of evaluating your illness, post-exertion malaise is part of the diagnostic criteria. We have to get your RER—your respiratory exchange ratio—above 1.1 and then I'll take you about thirty seconds past that, depending on how you're feeling," the doctor explains.

"I can do that. I already do that on my own when I ride my bike."

"Well, that may be hurting you, but I'll hold my judgment until after the results come back." Dr. Peterson stands up and leaves, then my mom and I walk out of the doctor's office and get some lunch.

* * *

We eat at a local coffee shop, and I stare outside at the towering pine trees around Lake Tahoe and the deep blue water beyond the shore. My mom is sitting next to me at a small table, her legs crossed and one hand holding her phone while she talks to my sister. Claire is calling from Alaska, where she's living for the summer. My mom catches up on her adventures and fills her in on my visit with Dr. Peterson while I eavesdrop on their conversation and eat a sandwich.

Once my mom is off the phone with Claire, and I've finished eating, we drive back to Dr. Peterson's office so I can do the exercise test. Then I walk into a large room with a treadmill and other fitness and medical equipment. The exercise physiologist, an athletic woman probably in her late-forties, greets me and starts to assemble some of the equipment. She has me begin with a respiratory test in which I breathe into a corrugated plastic tube, spewing out the contents of my lungs for the machine to measure.

"Nope, not good enough," the exercise physiologist says. "Keep breathing until I tell you to stop."

"But I couldn't breathe anymore. I had nothing left."

"You had something left," she insists. "The machine said you did."

Fuck the machine. And fuck this lady. She's tougher than you were when you taught boot camp classes. She probably teaches her own boot camp up here in the woods, some primal thing where they lift logs and boulders and shit.

"I don't understand," I say.

"Just exhale as long as you can, even if it feels like there's nothing left," she replies. "Then, whatever you do, don't inhale, okay?"

"Sure."

You do realize that you just agreed to asphyxiate yourself, right?

I exhale, then exhale some more, and keep exhaling. I'm still exhaling and now there really is nothing left in my lungs, and not just a normal nothing left; it's more of an *I'm going to pass out* nothing left. I hold my breath in the loopy, lung-burning headspace until it feels as if I'm no longer breathing, except I am, the machine says I am.

Seriously, fuck this stupid machine.

The exercise physiologist finally stops me, and I try to regain a normal breathing pattern as she prepares the equipment for the VO_2 max test. She takes her time attaching electrodes to my body, then places a breathing tube in my mouth. It's almost identical to the breathing device I used in the respiratory test, but this one has an extension that reaches to the treadmill.

I start to walk on the treadmill while the exercise physiologist controls the speed—first two miles per hour, then 2.5, and finally 3.3. It's taxing enough as it is, but then the treadmill begins to elevate. The exercise physiologist increases the incline to level six then twelve, and lastly, 13.5. I'm really struggling to keep up.

Shit, this used to be the warm-up before your workouts. Now you're spent after a few minutes.

My leg muscles are on fire, throbbing with pain and weakness. The tremors are starting too, reverberating across my torso. I need to sit down, but I can't stop. I have to finish this test. It's the only chance I have to figure out what's wrong with my body.

Taking her cue from the machine, the exercise physiologist finally stops the treadmill and I get off. We finish up, then I go to the lab next door for a blood draw. There a phlebotomist takes a dozen vials of my blood, and I return with my mom to the exam room to wait for Dr. Peterson. A few minutes later he walks in.

"How'd you do?" the doctor asks, sitting down and opening a folder.

"Good, I guess."

"Let's see," Dr. Peterson says, reading over the results. "You had an RER of 1.15, which means you had a conclusive test. We took you a little bit past your max. What happened—and this typically happens, as you know—is your volume of oxygen started to come back down. This means you had a pretty consistent response to exercise, and you are well conditioned, despite being sick as long as you have been. The test is essentially measuring you as a machine, because that's all we are—just machines—right?"

"Right." I chuckle and wait for the doctor to continue.

"Your O_2 pulse is thirteen milliliters per beat, and that is low—it should be eighteen. We usually see that in metabolic disorders." The doctor pauses and shuffles some papers around. "Now for your VO_2 max, which is what this is all about. The exercise test determines your level of fatigue. It was 28.6 milliliters per kilogram per minute, which is strikingly abnormal. Your body is very impaired. I do hundreds and hundreds of these tests on normal people your age, and that number should be in the forties, not 28.6."

"What does a typical CFS patient score?" I ask.

"Right around what you scored," the doctor answers. "A male with stage-four heart failure—you know, after a heart attack—has a VO_2 max of twenty, and you're just above that at twenty-eight. His problem is his heart won't pump; it's a different mechanism. Your problem is that your cells won't work."

"Oh," I say.

"Similarly, if I were to test a total couch potato, a man your age should score in the low thirties. You know this man, he's the guy you don't want to be—forty pounds overweight and drinks way too much beer. He would score around thirty-two milliliters per kilogram per minute or something like that. The difference is, you're sick and he's not."

"I see." I look at the doctor and nod.

"Now, in case you are wondering, the METs required for federal disability is seven, and you scored 8.2. So you would almost meet federal disability standards. I don't want you to focus on that. I'm just trying to put things in perspective," Dr. Peterson says.

"Okay, so don't aim for that?" I ask jokingly.

"Right, it shouldn't be your goal in life," he says. "This is not detraining, Jamison. This is not deconditioning. Please forgive me if you already know this stuff, but deconditioning would take you down three or four milliliters per kilogram on the test, okay? So maybe from a score of forty-five to forty-one, or something like that. That's after you've taken a few months off from exercise, which seems to basically be your case. This is a metabolic problem, Jamison. This is a mitochondrial problem." The doctor's voice takes on a dramatic tone. "You can't produce enough energy, and you're making yourself worse trying to do any kind of aerobic exercise."

"Really?" I'm not sure why I'm surprised. It's been obvious since the day I first got sick that exercise only makes my symptoms worse. I guess I was hoping it wasn't true, so I could ignore this whole illness and get back to bodybuilding.

"You can do limited resistance exercise, or try to, but light stretching might be best. When you do aerobic exercise, you're using very valuable energy, and just wasting it—pissing it down the drain. You should use it on something more productive, more lasting than sprinting on your bike. It would be better spent on a small outdoor project, or something like that."

"That's really hard for me. I would rather work out than do an outdoor project, or anything else." Sadness and nostalgia well up inside me, but I have to hold my emotions in. I can't break down. Not now. Not here. "Exercise is the thing I love most. It's a big part of what I want to do with my life. I miss it so much."

"I understand. You'll get back to it. I get people like you back to it," Dr. Peterson says. I believe him when he says I'll get back to bodybuilding. Dr. Gretchen made similar promises for my recovery, but that was over a year ago, and she ended up being wrong about a lot of things. Dr. Peterson, on the other hand, is a specialist, and he knows this illness well enough to give me an accurate prognosis. "For now, focus on what you *can* do. If you do exercise, as you know, you want to stay under your anaerobic threshold of 114 beats per minute. So if you do yoga, or light resistance training, keep your heart rate under that and you should recover faster."

"All right, I'll definitely do that," I say. The thought of working out again, even just light lifting, fills me with hope. It's been so long since I've had a good workout that I've grown cynical about that kind of recovery. But Dr. Peterson makes it seem possible, if not probable. I can almost feel the iron bars in my hands, the upholstery on the workout benches, the lingering sweat and cleaning solution filling the humid gym.

"Now," the doctor says, "what has caused this? I would assume you were healthy three years ago, otherwise you wouldn't have been a trainer, so I don't think you were predisposed to this illness. Yours isn't a genetic issue. Those are the people who are born tired and sick. This is an acquired impairment."

"That's good to know," I say. It's hard to comprehend everything Dr. Peterson is saying. Thankfully my mom is in the room taking notes, and I'm recording the appointment on my phone so I can go over everything later, when my brain isn't as foggy.

"This illness could be caused by a number of things," he says. "But I'm going to bet the virus is the culprit. The Epstein-Barr virus takes control of your mitochondria and uses the energy they produce to run itself. Because a virus can't produce energy alone, it has to hijack your mitochondria. This tells me that, right now, as we speak, you have a very active process going on inside your body." The doctor shifts around in his chair. "Maybe you were worse a year ago, but I don't think so. I think, probably, you've been about the same and your reaction, or your description, or something else, has changed—or you've modified your life to require less energy."

"Well, see, I disagree with that, because when I first got sick, walking was a challenge. My mom had to basically carry me to the car at one point." I look over at my mom. She glances up from her notepad, and a tinge of sadness flashes across her face. "Back then I wouldn't have been able to make it to your office. But now I'm doing better. I don't need help walking, and I can pretty much take care of—"

"Well, okay, you may be right," the doctor says, interrupting me. "In any case, you have a very, very significant physical impairment on a functional basis. What determines energy is three things: the ability of your heart to pump—and I already told you that was normal, okay?" Dr. Peterson looks at me and I nod. "Then there's your ability to oxygenate blood, which was normal throughout the test you just did. And finally, your cellular ability to use oxygen to create work—that is what is so impaired. If it was normal, I would have canceled all your labs and referred you to a good psychiatrist. This test proves that the illness is *not* in your head."

"That's really good to hear." I smile at the doctor, thinking about the stark difference between him and Dr. Gretchen. He's not blaming my illness on depression and anxiety from the car accident. He's not handing out antidepressants like candy. He's putting in the work to figure out the real reason I'm sick. To hear him confirm my belief that this illness is not in my head makes me feel relieved and validated—my illness is physical; my symptoms are real, not imagined. No amount of therapy or meditation or antidepressants is going to cure me. I need real medical treatments and Dr. Peterson can give them to me.

"Some people have a hard time getting news like this," the doctor says, "but when they think about it, they're actually relieved to know that they're not just lazy or depressed. I have tested literally thousands of lazy and depressed people, and they all have normal VO_2 max results." I shift around nervously, unsure of how I feel about the characterization he just made. I decide to ignore it and focus on the good news he has given me. "Let me just say, as a fitness trainer, you would have driven yourself nuts, because trainers don't understand this illness. They don't understand the physiological aspects of it."

"I *do* drive myself nuts," I say.

"Of course you do," Dr. Peterson says, smiling at me. "Now, you will probably have a difficult time recovering over the next few days. As you know, post-exertion malaise is a major feature of CFS. But I think you have almost no confounding issues going on. This is one illness. This is not eighteen different illnesses. And I hope you aren't surprised by these results, because you shouldn't be."

"I'm not, but it's good to have the numbers," I reply.

"You're right about that," the doctor says, looking down at a piece of paper. "Now, what gives you the generalized fatigue? It's every cell in your body. It's your brain, it's your ear, it's everything. But because the rest of 'the machine' works so well, you compensate in a certain way. You compensate in the sense that, like you say, you can get up and take a shower, or walk around the block. If you were my age and had this disease, you wouldn't be able to do that."

"Right," I say.

"Even worse, I have very, very disabled CFS patients who have a VO_2 max of six or eight, or something like that, and they literally would have trouble going from this room to the front desk," the doctor says.

My mom has been quiet for most of the appointment, but now she looks like she wants to say something. "So, what's your treatment plan for Jamison? Do you have one yet?" she asks Dr. Peterson.

"I don't know yet. We have to wait for the lab results. We'll go over them during the next appointment. But the good news is I *do* know how sick he is," the doctor says.

He knows how sick I am. It's the first time I've heard a doctor say that, and it feels damn good.

CHAPTER 26

My Lust-Filled Fantasy

July 24 – 25, 2012

It's been a month since my appointment with Dr. Peterson, and we're still waiting for some of the bloodwork he ordered to be processed. While we wait for the results, I'm focusing on other parts of my recovery, mainly trying to take care of myself.

However temporarily, I'm going to try to live on my own again. For the next few weeks, I'll be subletting a house from Rita and Stanley, friends of my mom's. Rita, an energetic soul with bobbed hair and a knack for dressing stylishly, has been close with my family since before I was born, and I've known her partner, Stanley, a slender man with thin gray hair, for several years now. Despite reaching retirement age, they both remain youthful and busy.

Their house is in Santa Cruz—a quaint beach community south of San Francisco, on the north end of Monterey Bay. I was born in the Santa Cruz Mountains and have had an affinity for the area since my mom and I moved away when I was in elementary school. Eventually I'd like to find a permanent place to rent in Santa Cruz, but right now I'm content subletting.

One condition of renting from Rita and Stanley is that I have to take care of Amy, their rather large cat. It's probably a bad idea, considering I can barely take care of myself, but it'll be worth it to have a place to stay near the beach.

When I first arrive at the house, Rita and Stanley have already left, and Amy is screeching for food. The instructions for feeding her are fairly simple: twice a day, once early in the morning and once in the evening. The instructions also stress the importance of feeding Amy on time, otherwise she will, like an angry child being carried out of a candy store, scratch and claw and make noise in every possible way until she gets what she wants.

After feeding Amy and unpacking my things, I get a text message from Sasha. I haven't seen her since I left Sonoma, and today she's in the area and wants to hang out. I scramble to make the house and myself look presentable. Then I hear a knock on the door and welcome her inside.

Sasha and I sit on the couch and talk. She tells me about her job and how she misses college, while I stare at her soft face and sweet smile. As she talks, my eyes drift down to her arms. They're toned and shapely, but something else gets my attention. Sasha's forearms are marked by scars, several thin horizontal lines of raised, pink tissue. I squint at them as if they're a complicated puzzle in need of solving

"What are you looking at?" Sasha asks, eyeballing me.

"Oh, sorry. I didn't mean to stare." I turn away, embarrassed.

"It's okay." She holds up her arm and rubs one of the scars. "I'm open about it."

"What happened?" I ask.

"High school was a dark time for me. Things are better now, but I guess depression always sort of sticks with you. Do you ever get depressed?"

"Sometimes, I guess." I don't want to talk about being depressed. After a year and a half of wondering if my illness was caused by depression, I'm still afraid that if I tell people that I get depressed, they'll think it's the reason I'm sick, even though Dr. Peterson said it's not.

"What's depression feel like for you?" Sasha asks.

"I don't know. It's not fun, but thankfully I don't get it that often." I pause and think of something else to talk about. "Hey, are you hungry?"

"Oh, um, yeah sure," Sasha says.

I go to the kitchen and make dinner, then we eat and turn on a movie. In the middle of the movie, Sasha asks to spend the night, which sets off a spark within me, and in her too, judging by the way she inches over to me on the couch. We are so close that it would be impossible for us to get any closer without holding each other. Both of our bodies are turned toward each other—my hip is right up against her leg and her arm is resting next to my shoulder.

This is my chance to lean in and kiss her. I want to, but I'm just not sure if I should. It might be my last shot though. If I don't make a move now, Sasha could lose interest.

My heart is racing and my breath is shaky. I can't do it. I can't kiss Sasha. Dr. Peterson's words are in my head—I could give her this illness. I can't risk that, and besides, I don't know if I'm even well enough to be intimate with her. It could make my symptoms worse. With all these thoughts clouding my head, I quickly excuse myself to go to the bathroom.

When I return to the couch, the movie has ended, and I suggest that we go to bed. But the way I say it sounds like I want to share my bed with Sasha. And I do, but it's not that simple.

She looks at me curiously, and I stare back at her. I want her so badly. I want to grab Sasha and gently kiss her lips, then rush into the bedroom and tear her clothes off until she's under the covers, naked and thrusting for me. I want her perhaps more than I've ever wanted anyone, a feeling only intensified by the fact that I can't have her. Buried under my lust-filled fantasy is the realization that I can't compromise her health, or mine, for a night of pleasure.

"Thanks for letting me stay over," Sasha says, looking at me like she wants to kiss me, which makes me wonder if she knows I want to kiss her. "I'm really glad I'm here."

"I'm really glad you're here, too." I take a gulp of air and look at Sasha in her big, blue eyes. Then, finally, I make my move. "Okay, let me show you to your room."

* * *

It's morning, my bed is empty, and pain is coursing through my body. I feel weak and dizzy, and my symptoms only get worse when I sit up. I don't know why I feel so bad. I went to bed early. I didn't drink. I didn't have sex. I didn't even kiss Sasha.

My phone says I have a text message sent from her at two in the morning. In the message she thanked me for letting her stay over and hinted that she wanted me to sleep in her bed. I didn't think our visit could get any more awkward, but now it has, and I'm nervous about seeing her. Do I act like we're just friends? Do I pretend she didn't send me a text message in the middle of the night?

Once I'm out of bed, I tiptoe past her room. To my relief, the door is closed. I relax a bit and continue, walking softly to the kitchen.

"Good morning," Sasha says, standing by the kitchen sink, sipping coffee.

"Oh, hi," I say, startled by her and trying to gather my thoughts. "How are you?"

"I'm good. You?"

"I'm okay." I walk over to the stove. "I'm gonna make eggs. Want some?"

"Yeah sure," she says as she settles into a nearby chair.

"Kale scramble sound good?" Sasha nods and I smile at her. It's a forced smile, though. The truth is I don't want to make a kale scramble. I want someone to make a kale scramble for me, so I can go back to bed and let this flare of symptoms pass.

Why don't you ask her to help you cook? Tell her you're not feeling well. Tell her you need to rest. Let her into your world. Be honest. She might just surprise you.

After cooking the eggs, I make Sasha a plate with some pesto on top. We sit outside and eat, enjoying each other's company, as much as two sexually frustrated people can. Then Sasha packs her bag and we say goodbye. I'm not sure when I'll see her again, but after last night, I doubt she's still interested in me. Right now I feel too awful to think about that though. All I really care about is going back to sleep.

* * *

An obnoxious scratching sound wakes me up. I look around the cold, dark bedroom where I've been sleeping, then roll over on the bed and hear the sound again. Maybe it's the wind outside or a device making noise in another part of the house. I sit up with one eye open and the other still clinging to sleep. There's only silence. I wait for the sound, but still nothing, as if the source of the noise is watching me, waiting until I go back to sleep. Finally I give up and lie down with a blanket over my head and try to recreate my last dream. But as soon as I do, I hear the noise once again. It sounds like someone ripping apart Velcro.

There's a large window across the room. I peek up at it and see Amy perched outside with one of her claws scratching the window screen. She continues to claw at the screen, the sound still nagging at my ears while I grab my phone and look at the time. It's three in the morning. I've been asleep for at least twelve hours.

Reluctantly, I decide to get up and feed Amy. The hardwood floor is cold and creaky as I groggily step across it, bumping into walls, doors, tables, and everything else in the house with sharp edges. Amy follows my every step until I open the door and let her inside. She quickly finds the bag of cat food on the floor, her tiny nose sniffing the air around it. I fill a bowl with the little brown nuggets, and Amy can barely contain herself. She aggressively bumps and grinds her large body against my calf like a horny high schooler at a coed dance. Then she struts over to a cardboard scratch pad and sharpens her claws, as if she'll need them to be extra pointy to fillet the Friskies in her bowl. For my sake, for the sake of all Earth's creatures, so the world will continue to spin, I walk outside and give Amy the bowl of processed animal fat and protein.

She crouches on the deck in the backyard and thoroughly sauces herself on kitty chow, then saunters off through the yard, while I stumble back to bed. Falling asleep again is difficult. After a few hours of mostly unsuccessful attempts, I wake up and return to the deck, where evidence of a feline feast is scattered about. Crumbs of cat food are sprinkled across the wood planks, the bowl is entirely empty, and there's a misshapen furry belly protruding from a nearby bush.

I join Amy basking outside as the sun comes up, slowly warming the moist air. It's peaceful and relaxing, but on days like today when I'm not feeling well, it's almost impossible to enjoy anything. The corrosive, acidic feeling in my stomach and the fatigue consuming everything I do only weakens my mental health. It's far too easy to feel disappointed about my life and forget my triumphs—how I've regained some of my strength and can take care of myself again. Instead, I focus on all the missed opportunities I've had while I've been sick. I could have been working full time and living in my own place by now, maybe even lifting heavy weights again and posing in bodybuilding competitions. But I haven't done any of those things in a year and a half. And as much as I want to feel good about the progress I've made, there's no doubt that I'm still sick, still trying to get my life back.

CHAPTER 27

Purge All the Bad Stuff

August 7, 2012

After a long road trip from Santa Cruz to Tuolumne, and then Tuolumne to Lake Tahoe, I'm back in one of Dr. Peterson's exam rooms with my mom patiently sitting across from me, her blue eyes illuminated by the sunlight streaming in through the window beside her.

Several minutes go by and the doctor walks in. "Good morning," he says, sitting down and looking at me. "So . . . we're having trouble finding the majority of your labs, but we did get some back—your natural killer cell function is low, you have intestinal dysbiosis, and your mycoplasma is positive. Now I know what's driving your illness, which is great because it's very treatable. I'm excited when I see that. It proves that I can make you well."

"That's great," I say. "What does it mean?" I've never heard of mycoplasma or intestinal dysbiosis.

"The intestinal dysbiosis means you're not absorbing nutrients, which limits what I can give you because it won't be absorbed. Basically food is going right through you," Dr. Peterson says. "Mycoplasma I can also treat; I'm always thrilled when I have a positive mycoplasma patient. It's one of the smallest known bacteria, and it's festering in your body as we speak. It fits perfectly—you're young and it's an opportunistic organism that is spread among young men and women. It's not the kind of mycoplasma that is spread through sexual contact; this kind is in saliva."

"Okay, so what are the treatment options?" I ask.

"Well, we are going to have to treat these things while we wait for the other labs. When you come back for your next appointment, we should have those for you. In the meantime, we are going to treat what we know." The doctor takes a breath and starts writing a prescription. "Now, this is very important: I would like you to get exactly what I prescribe, not what the pharmacist thinks is smarter, or cheaper, or whatever. Okay?"

I look over at my mom and she nods. "Okay, sure," I tell the doctor.

"Intestinal dysbiosis needs to be treated in a very specific way. I use hospital-grade drugs because they do the trick. It'll be amazing how good you feel. And I'm serious about that. What you do first with intestinal dysbiosis is you purge all the bad stuff." The doctor gives me a smile. "That means you're probably going to get nasty stools with blood in them. Then, we replace the bad stuff with medical-grade, balanced bacteria that belong in your gut, which are called probiotics."

"All right." I try not to think about bloody stools. Thankfully the doctor changes the subject to something more enjoyable.

"Given this, you should have a full recovery within a year—set your timeframe properly—you'll be back to lifting weights and doing all sorts of things."

When I leave Dr. Peterson's office, I'm beaming with hope from his prognosis—I should have a full recovery within a year. He says it all depends on taking the exact treatments he prescribed, so my mom and I drive to a local pharmacy to fill the prescriptions. The doctor is having me take Zithromax and Xifaxan, two antibiotics; carnitine, a supplement used to support energy production; and Valtrex, a drug used to treat viral infections related to Epstein-Barr. He insisted that I get the brand name version of the drugs, not the generic kind. The only problem is that I can't afford them. The pharmacist says that the brand name drugs are not covered by my health insurance and will cost thousands of dollars out-of-pocket.

Just a few minutes ago, I was riding high on the thought of recovering from this illness, now my hopes have been destroyed by the need for expensive medicine that I can't afford. The exorbitant cost of prescription drugs is certainly not a secret, especially for people with poor health, but this is the first time I've had to face the harsh reality myself. If I don't pay for the medications, I may never get better. But I'm broke. I make sixteen thousand dollars a year writing web content and have twenty-four thousand dollars in student loan debt, how the hell am I supposed to pay for a bunch of little pills that cost thousands of dollars? One of the antibiotics alone, Xifaxan, costs more than a quarter of my annual income. How is that even possible? Antibiotics are ubiquitous in the United States, the wealthiest country in the world. They should be cheap, or at least affordable, but these antibiotics are neither cheap nor affordable.

Unable to pay for the prescriptions, I leave the pharmacy empty-handed, feeling helpless and angry. My mom might be even angrier. She has pure rage in her eyes as we drive back to Dr. Peterson's office, speeding past the large log cabins and quaint Alpine shops in the affluent Lake Tahoe community. In the parking lot, my mom yanks the keys from the ignition, pushes her car door open, and storms inside to find Dr. Peterson.

After ten minutes of nervously waiting outside, imagining my mom shouting at the doctor until he's lying in a fetal position, I see her reemerge from the office with red cheeks, tears in her eyes, and a big bag of little boxes.

"What are those?" I look at the bag in her hand.

"Samples," she says, handing me the bag and wiping the tears from her face.

"They gave them to you?" I look inside the bag and inspect the tiny boxes.

"I got a little upset with them, and they gave me everything you need, pretty much cleaned out their supply."

"For free?"

"For free!" my mom says, the tension on her face finally relaxing.

It's days like today that make me realize how infinitely harder my life would be without my mom's help. Throughout my life, she has gone to incredible lengths for me, even when I haven't deserved it. One night as a junior in high school, I got drunk at a park with my friends and abandoned my mom's car, which she had let me borrow for the night. After the police brought me home, she got up early the next morning and walked across town to retrieve the car. I woke up a few hours later hungover and ashamed that she didn't make me get the car. But that's just her selfless nature—she doesn't have a punitive bone in her body, unless she's dealing with a doctor and pharmacist trying to bankrupt her son. Then she'll hunt their asses down.

I feel bad that my mom had to make a scene just to get the medicine I need, but I'm also glad she did. There was no way I could have paid for those medications.

Fuck these rich people with their fancy pharmacies and expensive-ass drugs. Shit, you could buy illegal drugs for cheaper. You could get a pound of cocaine for less than the cost of the antibiotics.

Standing outside the doctor's office, I swallow the pills with a few gulps of water and toss the bag of medications in the back of the car. Then my mom drives us south from Lake Tahoe toward Tuolumne while I recline my seat, cover my eyes with a hat, and try to think about getting better, not the ordeal that just happened.

CHAPTER 28

Soul-Crushing Revelations

November 20, 2012

I felt optimistic during my last appointment with Dr. Peterson. He did, after all, say I'd recover from this illness within a year. It seemed that, with his care, I would definitely get better. I still believe that I will, but I can't ignore the reality of the situation. For the last two months, I've been taking the medications he gave me, and there has yet to be any improvement in my health.

I'm going to give the treatments more time to kick in, but these long road trips to Dr. Peterson's office are beginning to take a toll on me. They're full of expensive bills, stacks of paperwork, monotonous phone calls with my health insurance provider, soul-crushing revelations at the pharmacy, and lots of time spent in the waiting room.

It's astonishing how quickly—less than two years, really—that my life has become consumed by these things. I want so much to return to the way it was before I got sick, when I didn't have to worry about my health. I want to flush all my medications down the toilet and delete the number of the insurance company from my phone. I want to forget what the inside of a doctor's office looks like. But most of all, I just want to know that everything is going to be okay, that *I* am going to be okay. Right now, I don't know that. I only know that I've been sick for two years, and it has made me depressed to the point that I've had some truly scary thoughts lately.

A few nights ago, I took Valtrex, along with the other medications that Dr. Peterson gave me, then I went to the grocery store with my mom and tried to walk around. But I was too weak and sick to my stomach to stay on my feet, so I retreated to the car. While my mom shopped, I sat in the car, staring out the foggy windows like a depressed zombie. The despair I felt made me think of the car accident—maybe the man I killed was dealing with depression before my car collided with his on the Napa River Bridge; maybe he was sick like me, maybe even terminally ill. For a moment, I could see myself parked in the middle of the bridge, waiting, wanting someone to end my life because I couldn't do it myself. I thought about that for a long time, probably too long. Then my mom got in the car, and I told her how bleak everything felt.

"I don't want to do this anymore, Mom," I said, looking at her across the center console. "My life can't become this—all this medical stuff. And it's not even helping. The medications aren't working. I'm not getting better."

"Oh, kiddo," my mom said. She looked concerned and scared.

"I can't live the rest of my life like this: going to see the doctor, constantly taking medications, calling the insurance company. I'm so tired of it." My eyes filled with tears, and I told my mom that I didn't know if it was worth it—living such a stressful life—or whether it would be better to not live at all, to not have to worry about my health, to not have to fix my broken body.

I didn't say these things lightly, but the words felt hollow. As hopeless as everything seemed, I wasn't going to kill myself. I couldn't. Even if I had nothing left to live for, I would be too indecisive to make such an irreversible decision. Most days I can't even decide what shirt to wear, choosing to end my life would be impossible. But my mom didn't know that. She thought, in that moment, I was capable of doing anything.

"You have to promise to tell me if you're thinking of harming yourself," she told me, tears sliding down her cheeks. I didn't mean to scare her like that, but I had to tell someone what I was feeling. I needed to talk about the darkness inside me.

* * *

After driving from Tuolumne to Lake Tahoe and staying in a hotel last night, my mom and I arrive at Dr. Peterson's office for another morning appointment. We sit in the waiting room, then in an exam room, and a few minutes later the doctor walks in.

"Hello, Jamison. How do you feel?" Dr. Peterson asks, moving across the room at an expeditious pace.

"I've been feeling pretty bad lately. It seems to be related to taking the Valtrex. I'd say I feel worse than I did at our last appointment."

"All right, but in what ways do you feel better?"

"I . . . I don't feel better. At all. I feel worse." At the risk of sounding like I'm complaining, I've decided to be blunt with the doctor.

"Okay, in what ways do you feel worse?"

"I've been a lot weaker. And I've had really bad nausea, a lot of stomach issues."

"Well, maybe your carnitine levels will be normal, and you can stop taking it, because that does upset the stomach. It shouldn't be the Valtrex."

"But as soon as I started taking Valtrex, I felt worse."

"Okay, well, the good news is your mycoplasma is negative," the doctor says, looking at my lab results. "As you may recall, it had a strong presence in your body, but it looks like we nailed that. It's a goner."

"That's great," my mom says, perking up on the other side of the room.

"That was my primary goal," Dr. Peterson says. "Of everything I was trying to do for you, that was it. Having gotten rid of the mycoplasma, you should now find yourself feeling better with more energy. Because of that, I will use a preemptive approach and take you off the carnitine supplement, unless you hear from me. That should make a significant difference with your nausea."

"There's something I need to mention," my mom says. "Jamison's level of depression has been pretty scary."

"Tell me about that . . ." Dr. Peterson says, looking at me.

"I would call it more than depression." I look at the doctor and try to find the words to express what I've been feeling. "It had a lot to do with the dive my health took. You know, because I was experiencing a certain quality of life that was pretty good compared to when I first got sick, and now it's devastating to slide back down. The weakness has been intense with so much pain and nausea—I mean, some days I can't even walk upstairs. It's just too much. I had been at a similar point, when the illness first started, and it was just miserable. So to be in that place again is—"

"A psychological hit," the doctor adds. "A fearful thing. 'I'm going to lose the ground I gained.'"

"Exactly," I reply.

"He would say stuff like, 'I've never felt like this,'" my mom adds.

I look at her, then at the doctor, and continue: "I've never been a depressed person. I've always been an upbeat, happy guy. So to be that sick and that depressed, it's like, man, this isn't my life."

My mom shifts around in her chair, looking at Dr. Peterson. "And he'd say things like, 'If I had the balls, I would . . .'"

"'Kill myself'?" the doctor asks.

"Yeah." I let out a long sigh and look at the floor. I'm ashamed I said that, especially to my mom. She didn't need to hear that, but I needed to say it.

"The fact that you talk about it is probably a good sign," Dr. Peterson says. "Because people who say that never do it. They're communicating, which is great. It's the people who don't say anything that I worry about. Now, I think I did something with you that I don't normally do. I put you on multiple drugs at one time to get you better faster. It's commonly not well tolerated. I made this decision because you are young, and otherwise healthy, and we needed to get through some of these steps faster."

"That makes sense," I say.

"I'm going to predict your labs are better now, and you're on the road to recovery. What you're experiencing is a lot of side effects from very, very potent drugs, especially for somebody who doesn't particularly take drugs. So it does make a lot of sense."

The doctor makes a good point—I've never been one to take drugs, of any kind, and my body usually doesn't tolerate them, so it's understandable that I'm having a bad reaction to the medications.

With the doctor's new orders to stop taking most of the medications, I leave Lake Tahoe, hoping that the side effects wear off and my health improves.

YEAR 3

False Hope

CHAPTER 29

A Fight That I Would Inevitably Lose

December 17, 2012

Once again, my mom is driving the Xterra, and I'm in the front seat. She recently bought the car from me because I'm rarely well enough to drive it, and I could use the money to pay for all my medical bills.

We're driving from Tuolumne to Santa Cruz, and since Rita and Stanley are no longer subletting their house, I'll be renting a cottage near the beach for a couple weeks, hoping the sea breeze and change of scenery will give my body a boost.

At Dr. Peterson's request, I've stopped taking the medications he prescribed. The depression has improved, but many of my physical symptoms have yet to get better. Today I'm feeling extra sick, sitting in a bubbling stew of nausea, with pain siphoning off my strength.

Before leaving town, we stop at a gas station. I stay in the car while my mom pumps the gas, checks the oil, washes the windows, and does other car maintenance. At the pump beside us is a teen who looks fresh off his learner's permit. He's checking under the hood of a lifted SUV from the early nineties that, by all indications, is older than he is. It's the type of vehicle that looks like the mud is actually part of the paint job. The guy, a kid really, keeps looking at my mom, then shifting his disapproving eyes to me.

"You have to do all the work, huh?" he says to my mom while she scrubs dead bugs off the windshield.

"Say again?" she replies.

"Looks like you have to do all the work yourself," he says, glaring at me as I rest my head on the passenger side window.

"Oh," my mom says, nervously.

The kid doesn't acknowledge her response, and instead looks directly at me, shakes his head, and says, "That's not right, just not right at all."

A rush of adrenaline surges through me. I want to get out of the car and beat him unconscious. But I won't. The physical repercussions of engaging with him would be immense. Even if I had the strength to confront him, which I don't, the exertion would surely make me sicker, and my intuition tells me that getting in a fight with anyone right now is a fight that I would inevitably lose. So I pretend I didn't hear what he said, even though I did, and his words are now gnawing at my ego. I'm angry because this ignorant, small-minded little man is a reminder of just how far my health has deteriorated, and how easy it is to feel insecure when challenged by a stronger, healthier person. Before I got sick, I would have defended myself against this punk, but living with a chronic illness has made me realize that I have to pick my battles.

He needs to mind his own business and to get his ass beat, but not by you—let someone else do it. Let the next person he spouts his immature mouth off to give him a beating. As much as you'd love to kick him off his high horse of distorted chivalry, everyone will be better off if you just pretend he didn't say anything. That fuck has no idea what your story is—he doesn't know that if you had the energy to fill the car with gas and wash the damn windows, you would, and then you'd walk over and ram the pump's nozzle straight up his ass.

We leave the gas station without incident, and the next hour of the drive is silent. I don't say a word. I'm too embarrassed, too frustrated, and too angry to talk about anything. Eventually my mom breaks the silence and apologizes for not sticking up for me at the gas station. I explain that my infirm body and consequential embarrassment was the reason for my silence. I tell her that I wanted to scream at the kid at the gas station, or better yet, pummel him with the squeegee, then wash the windows. But mostly, I just wanted to tell him that washing a car doesn't make you a better person, or even a stronger one; it doesn't make you anything except able-bodied, something he obviously takes for granted.

Like the amazing mother she is, my mom calms me down merely by being present. She listens to my frustrations, my anger, my sadness, as we continue driving. Around the halfway point of the drive, we come up behind a semi-truck holding up a line of cars behind us. The two-lane road makes passing the large truck tricky.

My mom slowly veers into the oncoming lane to check for clearance but retreats when two cars approach. She waits a couple minutes, then tries again, but more cars come. Finally she veers into the lane with only one car off in the distance. Then my mom stamps her foot on the gas pedal, and we speed along the rear of the truck. The car in the distance approaches. It's hard to tell how much road there is between us. It's going to be close. My foot slams down on the floor of the Xterra as if there's a brake installed on my side. I grab the armrest and open my mouth to say something, but only a groan comes out.

We have about twenty-five feet of the semi-truck left to clear, but the oncoming car isn't slowing down. My mom stamps on the gas once more, even harder this time, as we roar along the truck's cab. Then, with more grace than I could ever have, she steers the Xterra in front of the truck, and the oncoming car whizzes by.

I try to settle my nerves and slow my heart rate, but I can't do it while we're driving. I need to get out of the car.

"Hey, Mom, will you pull over?"

"Say again, sweetie?"

"Will you please pull over?"

"Oh, sure," she says. "Let me find a turnoff. Was that too close for you back there?"

"A little, but I'll be fine. I just need to stop for a bit."

We pull over and I walk to an irrigation ditch on the side of the road and sit on the loose gravel. To my left is a locked gate, and on the other side is a marsh where wind blows tall grasses in every direction and birds tweet to each other, oblivious of the man-made chaos a hundred feet away.

For several minutes, I stare blankly at the horizon, then my mom walks over and puts her hand on my back. My body is tense as she rubs my shoulder and apologizes for her aggressive driving.

"I won't pass any more trucks," she says.

"Ever?" I ask.

"Well, maybe just this trip," she replies, laughing.

"You're funny, Mom," I say, shaking my head. "It's fine. I'll be fine."

We get back in the car, the sun shining brightly through the windshield. My mom pulls down her overhead visor, and I notice something is missing. The laminated hospital bracelet is gone. I unpinned it from the visor and put it in a keepsake box before I sold the Xterra to my mom. Like an old, beaten, and discarded shield of battle, it had served its purpose and I didn't need it anymore.

Three years ago, the close call with the semi-truck would have left me scrambling to find the bracelet, questioning what was real and what was imagined, haunted by anxiety and nightmarish flashbacks. But now I've processed the trauma of the car accident to a point that I no longer need a piece of plastic to guide me. I can find my own way. And I will.

CHAPTER 30

Almost Normal

February 4, 2013

I've been off the medications for a few months now, and I'm feeling better. The side effects have stopped, and I'm finally making some progress again, which is why my mom and I are back at Dr. Peterson's office for a follow-up appointment.

The doctor walks in the room with a cheery smile.

"Feeling better?" he asks.

"Yeah, a bit better," I reply, smiling politely.

"What are you able to do?"

"My energy and strength are improving. Generally in the evenings I still hit a wall, but there's a good chunk of the day when I can get out and do stuff. I still have bad days. But on good days, I would say I feel sixty percent normal."

"Which is way better than you were."

"Yeah, definitely." I nod.

"And your stomach feels better?" he asks.

"Eh, kinda—it's still pretty funky. I'm not sure if that's because of something I'm eating, or if it's related to the illness." I look at the doctor for his input, but he doesn't say anything. "So, the lab results were . . ."

"Almost normal," Dr. Peterson says.

"Almost normal?" I ask.

"Yes, but I bet today they are completely normal." He looks at my mom sitting across the room. "Have you noticed improvements in him as well?"

"Yes, some improvement," she replies.

"I would hope so," the doctor says.

"I'm a little confused. When you say 'almost normal,' what do you mean?" I ask, looking at the doctor for more information.

"Well, as I mentioned last time, the mycoplasma is negative. So, we hit the culprit hard." The doctor turns to my mom again. "Doesn't he look great?"

"Yes," she says. "But will you tell us what his abnormal labs are?"

"Oh, they're just small things. Could even be an error." Dr. Peterson smiles at my mom. "I want to focus on how much better he looks. It's like he's a different man. I was thinking I should start doing before and after photos, because even patients forget. It really would be dramatic. They might think, 'Oh, I wasn't really that dysfunctional,' but they were."

Before and after photos? What is this? A reality show?

The doctor gets up from his chair and walks over to me with his medical tools in hand. Then he feels along my neck and underarms. "You have no swollen lymph nodes right now, none at all." He finishes the physical exam by listening to my lungs and heart. "How much exercise are you able to do? I know how important that is to you."

"Exercise is a struggle. It still makes me sick. I'll do some body weight exercises, a couple push-ups or squats, and it'll take me a week to recover. It feels impossible to build any level of conditioning."

"I know I don't need to teach you about physical exertion," the doctor says. "But you know to go slow from here, right?"

"Yes, I'm working on that. I've always been good at telling other people how much to exercise, but I've never been good at pacing myself."

"Well, you have to push only in small increments. You'll get back to those workouts again, you will. I think if your labs are normal today, I don't need to see you again. Okay?"

"Really?" I'm surprised, maybe even shocked, that Dr. Peterson thinks he doesn't need to see me again. It feels premature and a little dismissive, like he's made up his mind that I'm cured before I'm actually cured.

"Yes, if your labs are completely normal, you won't need another appointment," the doctor says, looking over my patient folder. "Your serotonin was at two hundred, which is perfectly fine, so your brain function should be getting back to normal as well."

"What if the labs aren't normal today?" my mom asks.

"I'm not sure. I'll come up with something. But I bet they'll be normal. So go for life!" Dr. Peterson says with an enthusiastic ring to his voice. "Before I go, do you have any questions? This could be your last shot at me."

"Oh, geez. Well, I still have a good amount of nausea and fatigue, and because everyone loves to bring it up, do you think gluten could be an issue for me?"

"I could test you for it now that you're better. It's a fad right now; most people aren't actually allergic to it. They may feel better not eating it because it does create gas, but I bet it has little to do with what you're experiencing," the doctor says.

"That's good, because I love gluten."

"Yes, well, it does make everything taste better," Dr. Peterson says. He pauses and looks down at some papers. "All right, well, I am very pleased with your recovery. Your testosterone is back to normal at eight hundred, so your libido and sex drive should be back to normal, too. It usually goes down when guys get sick, as yours did." The doctor shuts my folder and looks over at me. "All signs show you are out of the woods—your lymph nodes aren't swollen, your lungs are clear, your spleen isn't enlarged."

"So you think I will keep—"

"Getting better? Yes," Dr. Peterson says. "If you hit a wall, you should back off a bit. The first thing you should do is not a sixty-mile bike ride."

"Okay, gotcha."

"You'll be back to where you were in four to six months. Someone older would take much longer. Especially with your history of bodybuilding, you should recover quickly. I know I don't look like it, but I've lifted weights my entire life. Trust me—less is more."

"Before I got sick, I was doing the exact opposite. Every time I went to the gym it was like doing a marathon with weights. But that was my thing; I loved it. If I didn't hit the three-hour mark, it wasn't a good workout, you know?"

"I know. It's very common, and people get injured. You injured your immune system. That's something people don't think about. My son was a very serious bodybuilder in college. He worked at a gym and would see guys overtraining all the time, getting sick from all the germs and all the people," Dr. Peterson says, gathering his notes.

He wishes me well, then gets up, walks out the door, and just like that he's gone. He didn't tell me to call him if my symptoms get worse, or even to schedule a checkup in six months.

He just walked out, leaving me with an apprehensive feeling, as if I've been deserted, abandoned and left to fend for myself with an illness that, for all I know, is still ravaging my body. But because I want to be optimistic and because I want to believe that Dr. Peterson is right, I follow his orders and leave his office expecting to fully recover and never see him again.

As he said back in August, within a year I should be healthy and lifting weights. I may feel uncertain about my health and a bit skeptical of Dr. Peterson's prognosis, but if he's right and I recover without any further treatments, I will be genuinely thrilled, maybe the happiest I've ever been.

CHAPTER 31

Subletting

March 1, 2013

Rita and Stanley are on vacation and have again asked me to sublet their house and feed their cat, Amy. Every time I stay at their house, I'm reminded of how deceptively large the property is. From the street, the house looks like an ordinary home with a small backyard, but the lot is huge with three additional rentals on the property.

There's a small apartment attached to the main house, a secluded cottage on the back side of the lot, and a detached studio on another side of the house. Staying here gives me a glimpse of what it would be like to have a place of my own in Santa Cruz. I can imagine sitting outside every morning, a sea breeze drifting up from the beach, then riding my bike around the neighborhood, admiring all the restored Victorians and cozy beach bungalows. I would love that life and happily move into any of Rita and Stanley's rentals to make it reality, but right now they're all occupied.

I've looked at a few other places in the area, but Santa Cruz's rental market is ruthless, making for exorbitant rent prices and unlivable conditions. I recently looked at a small, dingy surf shack in someone's backyard. It was barely a step above a toolshed, with a hot plate, one window, and copious mold throughout. It all could have been mine for twelve hundred dollars a month, except there were twelve other prospective tenants on the waitlist in front of me.

Looking for a place to live is exhausting, and I don't want to use up all my energy, so today I'm lounging on the back deck, enjoying the cool breeze blowing up from the ocean. I start to drift off to sleep, but then I get startled by a woman walking through the backyard. She's dressed entirely in black—yoga pants, a long sleeve shirt, and a beanie. Even her ear-length hair is dyed jet black. Her smile, though, is bright and welcoming. She steps on the deck and puts out her hand.

"Hi. Are you Jamison?"

"Yeah. Hi." I sit up on the lounge chair and shake her hand.

Ask her for her name, you idiot. You act like you've never met someone before.

"I'm Lily," she says. "I rent the cottage in the back; it's my little *casita*." She lets go of my hand and tucks a few strands of hair behind one of her ears. "You're subletting for Stanley and Rita?"

"Yeah, but I'm hoping to find a permanent place soon."

"It's very competitive down here," she says. "I hope you can find a place."

"Thanks. Me too." I pause and think of how to keep the conversation going. "So, do you work around here?"

"Yeah, I'm a hair stylist," Lily says.

"That's cool. Do you enjoy it?"

"Most of the time, yeah, but I wish I could work outside more. Being stuck inside the salon all day isn't fun."

"I bet. Do you ever get to cut hair outside?"

"Sometimes, but not often," Lily says.

"You probably get this a lot, but would you cut my hair? I'll pay whatever you charge." Lily hesitates for a second. "We could do it outside," I continue.

"Okay. Sure," she says. "I don't usually cut men's hair, but I'll cut yours."

"When are you free?" I ask.

"Today I'm pretty much wide open. When's good for you?" Lily asks.

"How about this afternoon, around four?"

"Sounds good. Just knock on my door when you're ready," she says. Then she gives me a little wave and walks back to her cottage.

* * *

It's almost four and I'm staring at my phone, waiting until the last minute to go find Lily. If I walk slowly, which I'm sure to do, it will take maybe a minute to get to Lily's place. Finally I step off the deck and walk through the backyard—past the laundry room, a small water fountain, and two other rentals surrounded by lush plants and fruit trees.

Before knocking on her door, I stop to take in Lily's cottage. With a sunken roof and peeling paint, it doesn't look like much from the outside, but when she opens the door, it immediately feels homey and inviting. It's a warm, aromatic, and cozy little place. The floors are Spanish tile and the decor is eclectic, full of things you would find at a thrift store—a couch from the seventies and an old desktop computer collecting dust.

Lily welcomes me inside with a warm hug, then introduces her dog, a Pomeranian that is just as cute as her owner. So far Lily is a mystery to me, and in some ways, maybe even an anomaly. Her age is particularly hard to pinpoint. She doesn't look older than thirty, but as she's moving a salon chair outside to the garden, she casually tells me that she's thirty-four, almost ten years older than me.

After I'm settled in the chair, Lily grabs her scissors and goes to work on my hair. The sun shines on her tanned olive skin as little hair trimmings fall to the ground. I sit and ask about her past and her present. She tells me that she used to be married and lived in San Francisco, where she worked in sales for a beauty supply company, but the job and marriage didn't work out. She also tells me about her travels, tasting foods in foreign lands, making money, losing money, and eventually finding a home in Santa Cruz.

Lily has what I want: a little cottage in a charming beach town. I try not to let my jealousy show. I am, after all, just happy to be here, even if my stay is temporary. As Lily cuts my hair, her touch gentle and well-placed, I close my eyes and listen to the sound of air entering my lungs, the wind blowing through the trees, the buzzing of carpenter bees, the *snip* of scissors, and, of course, the clawing of Amy's scratch pad.

Peace is just that fleeting.

CHAPTER 32

What I Need

March 15, 2013

I've been so wrapped up in my illness, so consumed by trying to get better and, well, not getting worse, that I've lost touch with a lot of people, including my sister. Earlier today I realized that I forgot her birthday. It hit me like a slap upside my head. Thankfully she forgave me after I called and apologized. But I still feel bad, like a giant shithead, actually. I don't want to entirely blame my forgetfulness on the illness because I hate to use it as an excuse, but truthfully, brain fog is one of my most persistent symptoms. Just a few years ago, I had a sharp memory and never forgot important things like Claire's birthday. But now my brain is cloudy and full of lapses. Most days I can't even remember what I had for breakfast or whether I brushed my teeth.

Once I shake off my guilt about missing Claire's birthday, I carry on with the day. Then, awhile later, Lily comes over for dinner. We put together two plates with cabbage, quinoa, and asparagus soaked in olive oil and bring them to the couch. While we eat, the conversation flows nicely. It's a mellow evening. Even Amy is relaxed, curled up in front of the couch on an area rug.

When we're done eating, Lily looks at me curiously, like she wants to ask me something, which makes me want to run and hide. I can tell she's going to ask me about my past, questions I don't want to answer, topics I'd rather not talk about.

"You don't have to tell me if you don't want to," Lily says, "but Stanley said that you have an illness caused by depression from a car accident."

"He said that?" I ask, defensively.

"Sorry, we don't have to talk about it," Lily replies.

"No, it's okay. It's just that I do sometimes have depression, but my illness isn't caused by it."

"Oh, but you know mental trauma can have physical effects, so maybe they're related." Lily shifts around on the couch. "I remember being traumatized after seeing a dog get hit by a car. I felt physically ill and depressed for weeks."

"The dog died?" I ask.

"No, she lived. It just really shook me up."

"Was that when you were a kid?"

"It was a few years ago," Lily explains. "My childhood was relatively free of trauma, thankfully. I was mostly raised by my aunt. She was wealthy and took good care of me. It was a charmed upbringing. But then she passed away and left everything to my mom, who had a bad drug problem and squandered my share of the inheritance."

"That must have been frustrating," I say.

"It was, and it still is, but let's talk about something else." Lily points to a large canvas painting on the wall of two men deep in thought. "Oh goodness, I love this painting. Look at the way the light hits the canvas. It's so gorgeous."

"Oh yeah. I like that one, too." My eyes glance over the painting.

As if taking her cue from the lull in the conversation, Amy rises from the floor, yawns, stretches her limbs, and lets out a guttural sound, one a dying cow would make. Then she awkwardly squats and releases a stream of liquid shit on the rug. It's one of the most disgusting things I've ever seen—or smelled. I jump up, ignoring my impaired body and the urge to puke. I start to gag as I snap my napkin at the cat.

Amy runs for the back door, leaving a trail of foul-smelling brown liquid behind her, but the door is closed, trapping her inside. I stomp my feet at Amy and finally let her go outside, then return to the living room and begrudgingly clean up her shit. Lily helps, but the whole time it feels like I'm one whiff away from projectile vomiting and one scrub away from collapsing on the shit-stained rug. My lungs are burning, and I'm getting weaker by the second.

Finally we get Amy's sludge cleaned up, and I climb onto the couch next to Lily, the smell of cat shit and cleaning solution lingering in the air.

"Well, that was fun," I say, glancing over at Lily. She looks beautiful, her chiseled face and smokey eyes accented by the dim lighting. "So . . . what were we talking about?"

"We were talking about your health," Lily says. "When did you get sick? Was it right after your car accident?"

"No, it was almost two years after the car accident. I was coping pretty well with the trauma at that point." I take a deep breath and wish I had avoided the topic because now it feels like I have to explain myself. "My illness started with mono. I had it for months and never got better. I still haven't fully recovered, and I get exhausted ridiculously easily, especially after cleaning up cat shit." I chuckle. "But I'm getting better at managing my energy usage and pacing myself. Have you ever had mono?"

"Nope, never had mono. But I remember that friends in high school would get it." Lily pauses, seeming to retrieve something from her memory. "Stanley said you used to do bodybuilding in high school and college. Did you stop when you got sick?"

"Yeah, I had to. I can't really lift weights anymore," I say. "What about you? Do you work out?" I look at her toned arms and flat stomach. "You look like you do."

"Oh, thanks, I—"

"Sorry, that probably sounded like I was flirting with you."

That's because you were, dummy. You couldn't be more obvious.

"You mean you weren't flirting with me?" Lily asks playfully.

"Maybe I was." I grin sheepishly. "Are you flirting with me?"

Lily looks into my eyes and smiles, her gaze fixed and intense, sensual and full of anticipation, like waiting for a signal—a green light, an alarm clock, a starting gun. I don't know if Lily wants me to make a move, but I want to make one. I just don't know if it's a good idea. It's the night with Sasha all over again. I don't know if I can keep up, and then there's the main question looming in my mind—the reason I avoided kissing Sasha, the reason I haven't kissed anyone in two years—am I contagious?

I convince myself that I'm not. There's no way I will give Lily this illness. I would have given it to dozens of people by now through shared food and close contact. If I were contagious, everyone I know would be sick. I'm done letting this illness rule my life, at least this part of it. I've had enough abstinence, enough of the fear of kissing someone and getting them sick. I can't go the rest of my life without intimacy. I need to touch and be touched. I need pleasure and affection. I need kisses, and I need them from Lily.

She's still looking at me intently. The moment has turned into a staring contest, a standoff, a duel with no one pulling the trigger. Lily finally breaks her stare and snuggles up to me. I wrap my arms around her. Then, after several seconds of rapid heartbeats and shaky breaths, I carefully place my hand on Lily's warm cheek and, because it's what I need, I gently kiss her lips.

CHAPTER 33

Everyone Has Scars

March 19, 2013

Lily gets home from work and knocks on the front door. I welcome her inside and she gives me a hug, then makes her way through the house and out the back door to her cottage. A few minutes later, she returns holding the flowers I left in her kitchen earlier today.

"Are these from you? There was no card," Lily says.

"I don't know." I shrug and smile playfully.

"You're so sweet. Come here." She gives me another hug and strokes the back of my head. Then we kiss—oh, do we ever kiss. And not friendly kissing, either. This is full-on, obnoxious, Cary Grant kissing, with even more flair.

We take a break from the kissing, and Lily lights some candles. Soon the entire house simmers with the glow of candlelight and the anticipation of pleasure. We are, as it seems, skipping dinner and going straight to the bedroom, albeit with one stipulation.

"Hey, so, I need you to shave. Your face feels like sandpaper when we kiss," Lily tells me.

"Okay, sure. I guess it is pretty scruffy. Give me a minute." I walk into the bathroom and take out my razor. I'm a little irked by her request, but I make the concession because it seems that any sort of physical intimacy between us is now contingent on whether I shave my face.

When I return from the bathroom, Lily is in bed, peering out from underneath the comforter. She uncovers herself, revealing her toned body in a lacy bra and panties. I slide into bed next to her wearing only a pair of boxer briefs. I reach out to touch her silky skin, but my hands are cold and startle her. She rubs them together while we kiss. Then I feel along her hips, tracing the fabric of her panties with my fingers.

She stops me and has a troubled look on her face.

"I need to talk to you about something," she says.

"Okay," I reply, panicking silently. So many thoughts blitz through my head—did I do something wrong?

Maybe you were too aggressive. Or maybe it's something else. Maybe you got her sick. You could have given her the illness when you first kissed. It has been about a month since then. It takes about that long for the Epstein-Barr virus to develop and symptoms to show.

"This is sort of awkward for me to bring up," Lily says, hesitating. "Okay, I'll just say it . . . I had breast implants, but I took them out."

"Oh . . ." I glance down at her breasts, then quickly catch myself. "How long ago was that?"

"About two years ago."

"You didn't like them?"

"I hated them. They were too big—Ds," she says. "I became very self-conscious. I was constantly covering up my chest."

"It sounds like you made the right choice."

"Oh, yes, I definitely did. *Phew.* But when you see me naked, I just want you to know why they look the way they do."

"Hey, don't worry. You're gorgeous; you really are. I hope you know that."

"I'm not worried. I just want you to know what the scars are from," she says.

"It's okay . . . everyone has scars."

And the winner for cheesiest line in bed goes to . . . you, definitely you.

Lily looks gorgeous in the flickering candlelight as she leans down and kisses me. So far the experience has been fairly simple, but it's about to get more complicated. I'm filled with excitement, perhaps too much, as my mind passes the burden of arousal on to my sick body. Taking intimacy this far feels foreign, more so than past nights of foreplay with Lily. Although I've ended my kissing dry spell, I haven't had sex in two years, and I can't help but feel pressure to perform. This illness, and my consequential abstinence, have made me doubt my ability to have sex.

We continue kissing and Lily presses her body against mine while I take off her bra and gently run my hands over her breasts, feeling the soft scar tissue around them. I don't want to make her feel uncomfortable, so I move my hands down to her abdomen, then the coarse lace of her panties. My breathing can barely keep up with the arousal.

The atmosphere and energy in the room is erotic but draining. Part of me wants to forget about sex and just snuggle with Lily instead. The other part of me, the part that almost always prevails in these situations, wants Lily to tie me to the bed and have her way with me.

We continue to kiss and touch, then kiss some more. But I feel sick, weak, and full of nausea, like some poor kid hanging off the side of a roller coaster, puking on everyone as the ride roars down the track. Either that or I'm the one getting puked on.

My heart races, and the tremors start again. It's hard to look sexy when it feels like I'm getting zapped by a cattle prod every few seconds. I try to hide the tremors, or at least distract Lily from them by kissing her. I'm weak and in pain, but I can't stop. Lily would not be happy. She slides off my boxers. I pull away, for just a moment, to catch my breath. Then I pull down her panties and she gets on top of me, kissing my neck and rubbing my chest.

She straightens her posture and looks down at me.

"I know this is our first time together, but I feel a strong connection to you, and as we become more connected, I'd rather not have a barrier between us when we make love." Lily continues to look at me, the perspiration on her skin glistening in the candlelight. "I just got off my period, so now is a good time to not use a condom. But I need to know that I'm the only one you're going to be with."

All at once I'm conflicted—there's a sultry woman on top of me, both of us yearning for the ultimate dose of pleasure, but my sex drive is fleeing like a bandit, and questions of sexual purity and potentially life-changing consequences are whizzing around my head.

As much as I like Lily, I don't know if this is the right thing to do. I'm not sure if I care more about ending my abstinence or sharing a soul-touching experience with her. I don't want to make sex a conquest when it should be a shared experience, but it's hard not to be motivated by accomplishment when I've been deprived of something for such a long time. My mind doesn't know what to do, but ultimately my body does. Any reluctance I feel is overtaken by intense lust and desire.

CHAPTER 34

A Painful, Sloppy, One-Sided Affair

March 26, 2013

My head is pounding, my stomach is queasy, my muscles are throbbing with pain, and my conscience is plagued by a terrifying sense of doom. This is a post-orgasm hangover at its worst, and no matter how hard I try, I can't shake the terror I feel about last night.

Once Lily and I started having sex, it didn't go well. I lost control of my body like an inexperienced teenager. I knew I didn't have the strength or stamina to have sex long enough to make it pleasurable for Lily, and as embarrassing as I knew it would be, I kept going. In my mind, stopping would have meant defeat, and I wanted to feel pleasure, however selfishly, while I still could.

Less than a minute after we started, my body shuttered and convulsed, then went limp and felt like someone had beaten me with a tire iron. Instead of pleasure, I felt sick, and instead of a connection with Lily, I felt embarrassed and remorseful.

At first Lily didn't notice, or she pretended not to. She kept grinding on top of me, but eventually she saw my inactivity, stopped, and asked, "Did you come already?"

I didn't know what to say. I just closed my eyes and laid there with a burning body, bruised ego, and an undeniable feeling of shame. And not just because I couldn't perform. I've had other sexual misadventures while I've been sick, but now that my health has improved, I'd hoped I could transcend those bad experiences. I couldn't.

Any uncertainty about the status of my health is now clear—I'm still sick, still waiting for Dr. Peterson's promise of a full recovery to be fulfilled. He told me that my testosterone is normal. I should be able to have sex like I used to. But I can't. Sex is still a painful, sloppy, one-sided affair that is barely worth the trouble. It's complicated enough for a healthy person; as a sick person, it's nearly impossible.

My other attempts at pleasuring Lily haven't gone much better. When I use my hands, they ache and burn with pain, and I usually have to stop. Of course, I can't bring myself to tell her this. Even if I could get over the humiliation, I'm not sure she'd understand.

I don't know if I'll ever have the courage to tell Lily what sex is like for me, or what it does to my body the next day. But right now there's something more pressing on my mind: I'm afraid Lily is going to get pregnant because we had unprotected sex.

Last night, during our foreplay, we hastily agreed to not use a condom. Today it seems that was a bad idea. The thought of supporting a child right now, physically and financially, is scary. Not because it's something I don't want, but rather because it's something I can't do. I can barely take care of myself; there's no way I could care for another human being. Even with Lily's help, I would hold myself to a standard of parenting that I just couldn't live up to while fighting a chronic illness. It's a heartbreaking realization. I've always imagined myself having children. Now that illness, and time, have stunted my ambitions, having kids feels unobtainable. Like many of my other aspirations, I have to suppress my desire to be a father and, in the process, bury my sorrow deep within my overloaded psyche. For me, right now, it's the only way to move forward.

Before getting out of bed, I search online for "unprotected sex ovulation cycle," and find that, as Lily said last night, our timing did reduce the odds of her getting pregnant. But it didn't eliminate the possibility of it happening. Anxiety consumes my thoughts as I prop myself up in bed.

Oh man, you're screwed. What if she gets pregnant? If you think life is difficult now, imagine raising a child while you're sick. That would be a nightmare.

The clock on my phone says it's around noon. I get up and walk to the kitchen where Lily is reading with a cup of tea in front of her.

"Hey there. If you want tea, there's hot water in the kettle," Lily says, sitting up in her chair and pointing to the stove. "I hope you don't mind that I made myself at home."

"Oh, please, make yourself at home. It's not mine." I laugh perhaps a bit too aggressively.

Then, with some hesitation, as if she's been thinking about it for hours, Lily asks, "So how do you feel about last night?"

"It was really special, and I'm glad I was able to experience it with you. It's just . . ." I'm trying to bring up my concerns about last night without seeming like a complete asshole, but even to my own ears, I sound like a phony politician.

"It's just . . . what?" Lily asks with a sharp tone.

"I guess I'm a just a little worried because we didn't use a condom."

"Oh, you are?" she says.

"Yeah, obviously you know more about it than I do, but I read that you could still get pregnant."

"I guess we did take a risk." Lily frowns. "Well, I have Plan B medication. Would you feel better if I take it?"

"Not if you don't want to; I know those things can be pretty unpleasant."

"It would basically just be restarting my period artificially. If you'd feel better, I should do it. I'd feel better, too."

"Okay, but I would like to make up for it somehow."

"Sure. Take me out to lunch?" Lily says. I smile and nod. Then we hug and kiss, and she goes off to find the medication while I take a shower and get dressed.

* * *

The physical and emotional consequences from last night linger in my body, leaving me weak, in pain, and feeling out of sorts. I should probably be in bed resting, but Lily took her dog for a walk, and now I'm driving around the neighborhood looking for her so we can go get lunch. Even on a good day with no sex hangover, I rarely feel well enough to drive, and today the sights and sounds of the busy Santa Cruz streets are really doing a number on me. But I'm not having any flashbacks to my car accident, so at least there's that.

After driving around aimlessly for several minutes, I find Lily and her dog. The Pomeranian is stoked by activity as Lily strolls happily behind her. They get in the car and I immediately feel like a sober person arriving late to a college party. Everyone is exuberant and having fun, except me.

We drive to the Harbor Café, a popular restaurant in Santa Cruz. It's packed, as usual, so we try the Windmill Café, a little coffee shop perched above Schwan Lagoon, surrounded by lofty palm trees. Most of the nearly century-old building looks like an ordinary café with a pointed roof and wood exterior, but the front also has a white, four-bladed windmill sticking out of it.

We order our food and sit outside on the patio as the sun warms the air between heavy clouds. Lily tends to her dog with treats and gentle kneading, while I enjoy the salty air rushing along East Cliff. Then Lily grabs our food from inside and brings it to the table.

"Aw, isn't this so lovely?" she says, looking around at the scenery.

"It really is. Thanks for suggesting it."

"My pleasure, sweets. Glad we could be here together."

"Me too." I smile while Lily sets a bowl of water on the ground for her dog. Then she sits up in her chair and looks at me like she just remembered something important.

"Oh," Lily says. "I've been meaning to tell you . . . I think you should give Amy better care."

"What do you mean?" I ask, trying not to sound defensive.

"I just noticed that her bowl was getting low on water, that's all," Lily says.

If she's so concerned, why doesn't she fill the bowl?

"Is that it?" My voice is snippy. So much for not being defensive.

"No, actually, it's not," Lily says, wielding her own attitude. "Amy is a living thing. She deserves good care."

"Good care?" I scoff and throw up my hands. "I feed her every morning before dawn. I cleaned her shit off the rug. How can you say I don't take good care of her?" My heart is thumping and I'm out of breath. I try to calm my body, but sitting next to Lily just makes me angrier. "I can't believe you're criticizing me about this. I'm pretty sure her bowl still has water in it, and there are two other water bowls around the property. It's not like she's dying of thirst."

"It was just my opinion." Lily shakes her head. "I need to be able to express my opinion."

"Yeah, well, I need to express when I think your opinion is ridiculous."

I turn away from Lily and try to think about anything other than pets and bad sexual experiences as we finish our meal in silence.

CHAPTER 35

Bone Broth

May 15, 2013

My relationship with Lily hasn't been going well. We've been arguing a lot lately and, against my better judgment, I'm now staying with her. After subletting from Rita and Stanley, I moved on to house sit for my cousin who lives a few blocks away, but one night Lily came over and found large patches of mold on the walls. Since then she has insisted that I stay at her cottage.

For a brief time it was a good situation. I thought I had finally found a place I could settle into with a woman I could love, mostly because Lily has an innate ability to nurture. She has gone shopping for me when I've been too sick to do it myself and given me massages when my muscles ached.

We've had a lot of enjoyable times together, meditating outside in the garden and going for scenic drives along Monterey Bay. But now those good times have become more infrequent, and the endearing feelings I once had for her have faded and turned to tension and acrimony.

Lily and I fight almost every day, a pattern that has existed between us for weeks. Some days the fighting starts with little jabs at each other's psyches, like when she gives me a territorial look as I walk around her cottage. Other days it's more obvious, like when Lily blames the clog in the bathroom sink on my beard trimmings, even though I use an electric razor that captures the shavings.

Maybe our egos are clashing, or maybe we're just not a good match. Maybe we've never been a good match. She's a lot older than me and has always treated me more like a younger brother than a partner. For my part, I've shied away from difficult conversations and haven't always been truthful with her about my health. Whatever is causing our strife, I feel bad about it. I feel bad that we're not getting along. I feel bad that I can't fix our relationship. And most of all, I feel bad that, at this point, there's only one reason I haven't ended the relationship: I need a place to stay.

If I break up with Lily, I'll have to go back to my mom's house in Tuolumne. And while I don't want to live with Lily anymore, I do want to stay in Santa Cruz. Unfortunately living with her is my only viable option until I find a place of my own.

I'm trying to be honest with myself about the living arrangement and my relationship with Lily as a whole, but I don't know how to be honest with her about either. I don't know how to tell her that our relationship isn't working and, at the same time, ask if I can stay in her cottage until I find somewhere else to live.

Not breaking up with Lily because I need a place to stay is far from my proudest life decision, but it's not like I'm free-loading. I pay half of her rent and utilities, and I buy all my own food. The rest of our living situation doesn't make me feel good, but hopefully I can get my own place soon so we can both move on.

For now, I get most days at the cottage by myself while Lily works. I cherish most of my time alone, except today because there's a rotten smell filling the entire cottage, wafting over the countertops in the kitchen, down the hall, and into the bedroom where I'm writing an article, however ironically, on successful relationships.

It's hard to concentrate with the smell of a dead animal swirling around me. For ten minutes, I comb through the kitchen trying to find the source. It's not the trash, not the compost, not my feet. Eventually I give up and go back to writing.

An hour later I emerge from the bedroom and the smell is just as strong. As an escape, I go for a walk, leaving the front door open to air out Lily's cottage. I step onto Cayuga, a road wider than most other residential streets, then turn left. At the corner of Broadway and Seabright, I stop next to a soothing water fountain in front of the Pacific Cultural Center. Then I turn left again and see the terracotta roof of Gault Elementary on the right. I'm only halfway around the block and already running low on strength, my muscles throbbing with pain. As miserable as I feel, it's still nice to get out and see the neighborhood. I spend so much time indoors that even touring the surrounding streets is a refreshing change of scenery.

My head starts to spin and I feel like vomiting, but I still want to finish the walk. I have to—turning back now would mean walking the same distance as finishing the loop around the block, and stopping to rest in front of some random person's house would surely set off alarms.

You can do this. You can walk a block. For fuck's sake, it wasn't that long ago that you were sprinting several blocks before lifting hundreds of pounds at the gym. Finish strong. You're almost home. Then you can rest.

I make a left on Effey and walk back to Cayuga, where I can see the path leading to Lily's cottage. Finally, I shuffle past the wooden gate, along the side of the main house, and through the open door of the cottage.

When I step inside, the awful smell is still there, and it only gets worse as I sit on a stool in the kitchen to catch my breath. To my left is a large pot sitting on the stove. I move closer and open the lid to find rotting cow bones soaking in a murky broth, which only increases the putrid smell in the air. Now I remember that Lily made the broth the other day. I don't know why she left it out, but I decide to leave it alone in case she wants to use it for something.

* * *

After lying down for a nap, I wake up and get out of bed. The sun has set and my walk around the block has caught up with me. Standing is difficult, so I kneel on the floor and shuffle over to my bag of clothes on the other side of the bedroom. Then I change into pajamas, stand up, and walk to the kitchen.

As soon as my feet hit the tiled floor, I get disoriented and lean on the stove with the pot of rotting bones and its rancid smell a few inches from my face. I uncover the pot again but then gag and abruptly cover it back up. I want to take the pot outside, but it's Lily's kitchen and I don't want to mess anything up. Plus, I'm not sure if I have the strength to carry a heavy metal pot full of bones and two gallons of broth, so I leave it on the stove and collapse on the couch.

Then I hear the entrance gate shut like two wood blocks slapping together. Anxiety rushes through me—someone's here. Lily's here. She walks in looking beautiful in a striped sundress, but she also seems tired and agitated.

"What's that smell?" Lily asks, a look of disgust on her face.

"I've been smelling it all day. I think it's the bone broth on the stove."

"*Yuck*," she says, sniffing the pot and carrying it outside.

"I wasn't sure if you were using it for something."

"What would I use rotten bones for?" Lily walks back inside with the empty pot and puts it in the sink.

"I don't know. *You* left them out." I retreat to the couch to conserve energy for what is sure to be another argument full of thinking and yelling and other things I should do sitting down, if at all.

"I don't understand what you were thinking," Lily says, her face flushing.

"What I was thinking? I'm not the one who left the pot of decaying bones on the stove." I shake my head. "I mean, what did you expect me to do?"

"Throw them out!" Lily shouts. "Get rid of them. The broth had obviously gone bad. The bones were rotting. You were here all day while I was at work, and it only would have taken you a few seconds to dump them out. But you didn't. You didn't do anything."

She knows you're at a disadvantage. She must know you don't have the strength to raise your voice as loud as hers. She's not going to take it easy on you. You need to stick up for yourself.

I stand up and want to shout back at her but get dizzy and feel like I might throw up, so I sit back down on the couch and speak as firmly as I can without raising my voice or puking.

"Let me get this straight. Without saying anything, you expected me to dump out the smelly-ass cow bones you left sitting on the stove? The same cow bones that smell like shit even when they aren't rotting? Doesn't that seem a little unreasonable to you?"

"No. It doesn't," she snaps. "It's common sense."

"You know what, I'm exhausted. I can't deal with this."

"I'm exhausted, too. I've been *working* all day," Lily says with a condescending tone.

"Oh, and I haven't been working?"

"I don't know what you've been doing. You've been at home. I haven't."

We are two otherwise pleasant people bringing out the ugliness in each other. Lily reams me about not buying dish soap and toilet paper. I bring up my contribution to her rent and the household items that I've paid for. The argument gets even more petty when she says I should have paid for her meal the last time we ate at a restaurant.

I've finally had enough. Her complaints become too much for my foggy brain to process. I give Lily one hundred dollars for her grievances, then leave. It is, at last, the end of our relationship.

CHAPTER 36

———

Relax the Body

September 15, 2013

Finally, after months of searching, I've found a place of my own in Santa Cruz. It's a two-hundred-square-foot studio converted from an old garage on Rita and Stanley's property. Shortly after I broke up with Lily, the studio, which is next to hers, opened up and I moved in. That's right—my ex-girlfriend is now my neighbor. It's not an ideal situation, but I'm grateful to have a place to live.

The studio has a bathroom, a kitchen sink, and a hot plate. It isn't much, but I've been wanting to permanently live on my own again for a long time, and this is my chance. I think it's going to be healthy and recuperative for me—a catalyst for recreating the life I had before getting sick. And while it's already been a good change, it has also come with complications.

Moving day was a struggle. I loaded my things into the Xterra at my mom's house with triple digit temperatures swirling around outside. It was about all my body could handle. I quickly curled up in the front seat while my mom drove through the Central Valley, one of the hottest parts of California. Then, a few hours later, we finally arrived in Santa Cruz with a cool ocean breeze on our faces.

It felt good to be in my new home, but soon the reality of living next to Lily started to sink in. The back door of my studio is only a few yards from her cottage, and she always seems to be walking around outside. For the most part, I've managed to avoid interacting with her, but it's impossible to avoid all of my neighbors. The front of my studio is practically touching Rita and Stanley's back deck and, when I have my blinds open, anyone can see inside from almost anywhere on the property.

It doesn't help that Rita and Stanley zip around my studio all day gardening and working on projects in their backyard. They try to respect my privacy, but like many people I know, they don't understand my illness. The other day, Rita came by my place, saw me resting in bed, and asked, "Do you sleep all the time because you're bored?"

She might as well have asked Michael J. Fox if his hands tremble because he's scared. I wasn't resting by choice. Resting is like pulling teeth for me. But it's what my body needs. If I were healthy and bored, I wouldn't be sleeping this much; I'd be lifting weights, going for a hike, or finding fun in other things I used to do before I got sick. Rita doesn't understand that most days I don't have the energy to even walk around the block.

She does help me in other ways though. She lets me borrow her car when I'm well enough to drive, and when I'm not, she brings me food and other items I would normally get for myself from the store. Maybe that's why it's so perplexing that she questions my need to rest. Comments like hers get under my skin and ultimately push me to do things I shouldn't, things that even Dr. Peterson said I need to avoid, things like exercise.

Today I've tricked myself into thinking that I'm well enough to train my first fitness client in three years. The training session will be entirely online through video chat, so I don't have to worry about getting myself to a gym or my client's house. All I have to do is conserve my energy, open my laptop, and wait for the client to appear on the screen.

I committed to doing another training session tomorrow, which, depending on how today goes, may have been a mistake. But exercise has been absent from my life for such a long time that I'm hoping these virtual training sessions will reintroduce it in a healthy way, one that will continue as my health improves.

You also need the money. You can make more from one training session than you do writing five of those shitty articles about relationships and portable toilets. You're living off food stamps and barely covering your rent. If you don't get more income soon, you can say goodbye to Santa Cruz and living on your own.

Once I'm out of bed, I set up my laptop, unroll a workout mat on the floor, and take out a whiteboard showing a list of the exercises that my client will be doing. Then I change into workout clothes, filling my mind with nostalgia and fond memories. Rummaging through my old gym bag only brings back more memories of bodybuilding and the days when I would hop on the Univega and ride to the gym. The bag is full of knee wraps for squats and leg presses, lifting straps for deadlifts and back exercises, and a sack full of chalk for gripping weights. I miss these things, these instruments of blissful torture. But I don't have time for nostalgia right now, I have to get ready to train my client.

After sitting down on my workout mat, I adjust the laptop on a chair in front of me and try to calm my nerves by meditating using the mantra: *relax the body, smile.* But I can't relax my body, and my smile feels more like a grimace.

Try again. Relax the body, smile.

I pick up my phone and look at the clock.

Put the phone down. Relax the body, smile.

The clock says it's just after five in the evening.

Stop looking at your phone. You have plenty of time. Relax the body, smile.

I reach over and tap on my laptop to make sure it's still working. Then I log into the video chat and check the connection—the screen is black. This could be bad.

For fuck's sake, it's fine. The screen is black because your client hasn't logged on yet. Be patient, relax the body, smile.

I'm worried that I won't be able to keep up with my client, that she'll see my shrunken muscles and know how out of shape I am—that my body is now soft and withered where it used to be firm and muscular, that I haven't worked out in three years and I spend most of my days horizontal in bed, living vicariously through my Netflix account.

She won't care. Relax the body, smile.

If I start feeling extra sick and have to stop the session, then she will definitely know something's wrong.

That won't happen. It'll be fine. Everything will be fine. Relax the body, smile. Relax the body, fucking smile!

A woman's face appears on the laptop's screen. The video quality is poor, but it looks like she's in her thirties with an angular face and short dark hair.

"Where are you streaming from today?" I ask.

"I'm in New York. Where are you?" she replies.

"California, near San Francisco. What time is it in New York? Around eight?"

"Yep, either now or early in the morning is the only time I have to work out," she explains.

"Well, good for you for getting it in when you can." I smile at the screen. "Okay, let's get started . . ."

To begin, we do bench dips, a triceps exercise, which my client does on a coffee table in her living room. Then we do overhead extensions, another triceps exercise that is usually done with resistance, but we both seem to be content without the added weight. Even so, conserving energy during an exertion-packed half-hour workout feels impossible, like trying to chew food without tasting it, or standing in the rain without getting wet. Conserving energy is especially difficult when I still hold myself to the personal and professional standard of always giving as much effort as I can.

After doing push-ups, kickbacks, leg lifts, and bicycle crunches, I take a break and look at my phone. There are only a few minutes left in the session. In a fraction of the time it used to take me to do a workout, I'm absolutely drained, and I barely did any of the exercises. For the remainder of the session, I check in with my client and ask her for feedback. She enjoyed the workout and wants to do more sessions, but regularly putting my body through this much pain and stress seems like a bad idea, and not just because I don't know if my body could handle it. From now on, my client's schedule only allows her to work out during a small window of time at three in the morning here in California. Yet, for some reason, some idiotic reason, I tell her that we might be able to make it work, since I'm usually awake at that hour.

Wait . . . What? When the hell are you awake at three in the morning? This is how you got sick in the first place—you over-extended yourself. There's no way, absolutely no fucking way you are going to train this client in the middle of the night. It doesn't matter how healthy you think you are, you're creating a fantasy, and it's not a good one.

Thoroughly exhausted, I close my laptop and sit on the floor, thinking of what it will be like to do this all over again tomorrow with a different client. I will probably do the same routine with the yoga mat, the laptop, the workout clothes I never wear, and my frantic attempt at pre-workout meditation. My eyes will eventually open, but the screen will again still be black, and then suddenly my client will appear. We'll do the same workout that I did with the client from New York, and toward the end of the thirty-minute session, I will feel the repercussions of doing two workouts with a sick body. Seconds away from shutting the laptop and crawling into bed, I will realize that I may have done too much. But I'll be okay with that. Like the workouts of my past life, I will just be happy to have lived it, happy to have moved and felt and experienced, all while teetering on the knife edge of extreme exhaustion and profound pleasure, not knowing what will happen next, and concluding that if it is indeed too much for my body, then so be it.

CHAPTER 37

Regression

November 28, 2013

My health has been declining a lot lately, and now I'm back at my mom's house in Tuolumne, trying to recuperate. I felt okay in September, even after training a couple clients on video chat, but now I'm significantly worse—weaker and more fatigued.

As I climb the stairs to the second floor of the house to take a shower, I'm reminded of just how debilitated my body can get with this illness. Three years after I got sick and first struggled to climb these stairs, I find myself doing the exact same thing, except now it's even more difficult. To get upstairs, I have to sit on the first step, then lift my body up to the next step, using my legs as traction. Each step takes a series of movements with its own set of challenges that deplete my muscles of what little energy they have. It feels like someone gave me too many muscle relaxants and then asked me to carry a one-hundred-and-sixty-pound bag of meat and bones up a flight of stairs.

I push the old bag of meat and bones up fifteen more steps, with long breaks in between. It takes me about an hour to get up the stairs, take a shower, and scoot my ass back down. It's a considerable chunk of my day, and shows that, even to my stubborn mindset, I'm not doing well.

It's hard to pinpoint exactly when my condition started deteriorating, probably because there's an ebb and flow from one day to the next, but in hindsight the difference is undeniable and substantial. When I first moved into my studio back in July, I could still walk around the block and, on good days, even ride the Univega a mile or so. Now walking to the bathroom is a major accomplishment, simple chores like washing the dishes have become arduous, and it feels like I'm always on the verge of vomiting.

Since I last saw Dr. Peterson almost a year ago, I've trusted that my health would continue to improve, but now it's clear that it hasn't. It's as if I had been slowly improving, or at least not getting worse, then a giant hand came along and swatted me down. This regression is why, after moving in only a few months ago, I've had to sublet my studio in Santa Cruz. I'm just not healthy enough to work and take care of myself. So until I regain the ground I've lost, I'm staying with my mom, who takes away much of the burden of cooking and other chores I struggle with. It feels like déjà vu though, like we've been in this situation before, probably because we have, several times.

It's beyond frustrating—enraging, really. I shouldn't be this sick. I shouldn't need my mom to take care of me. If Dr. Peterson's prognosis were correct, I wouldn't be reduced to going up and down stairs sitting on my ass. It's now apparent that he was wrong to say that I would recover in a year. His words now seem hollow, an empty promise, a guarantee he couldn't keep. I don't know why he wanted to stop treating me. Perhaps he was just trying to get rid of me—maybe he was scared of my thoughts of suicide or, more likely, my fierce mother who stormed into his office in search of affordable medications. Whatever Dr. Peterson's reason was for discontinuing my treatment, he wasn't upfront with me. And, to be honest, I'm pissed about it—furious that this illness and the universe have conspired to keep me sick, and angry at Dr. Peterson for making me believe that I would get better, and then, when I didn't, leaving me without proper medical care.

In the midst of my angst about not feeling better, I went online and found a YouTube video of Dr. Peterson being interviewed by journalist Llewellyn King. In the interview, which was posted several months before my last appointment with Dr. Peterson, King asked the doctor whether, in his twenty-five-year clinical career, he had ever seen a patient fully recover from chronic fatigue syndrome. Dr. Peterson responded by saying, "I don't think I've ever seen a full and total recovery. I've seen two things: I've seen people with substantial improvements to the point that they resume near normal lives, and I've seen people who have just come to grips with their symptoms and just get along, and continue moderately impaired, but they've adjusted their lives."

Dr. Peterson promised me something he had never seen. Based on his responses in that interview, he gave me a prognosis that was in direct conflict with every other case he had witnessed in the last twenty-five years. He shouldn't have done that, and as angry as it makes me that he did, I must accept the fact that he made a bad decision—that all doctors sometimes make bad decisions.

No doctor wants to admit that they've never seen a patient recover from an illness. Statements like that could cause patients, and the general public, to question the doctor's efficacy. But it could also serve as a real, human moment. Doctors are people who come with flaws and make mistakes just like everybody else, but society holds them to almost impossible standards. When they meet those extremely high standards, they are given a god-like status that can lead people, especially patients, to accept everything they say as fact. And sometimes it all works out—when they're right, everything is great—but the flip side is an ugly truth: it's easy for a doctor to pretend that they have the answer to someone's health problem, even though they don't.

When a doctor takes a patient down the wrong path, it can waste months, if not years, of that person's life. The doctor thinks they know the problem, treats it, then deems the patient well again, despite the illness still being active. For a while everyone is optimistic—the doctor thinks the treatment was successful and, although the patient still has symptoms, it seems as though everything will be better soon. That, of course, is what happened to me. And I'm just now pulling the veil off what my doctors have told me. Dr. Gretchen thought my illness was caused by depression from the car accident; Dr. Peterson thought treating mycoplasma would make me better. They were both wrong. And now I'm left feeling as confused as ever about my illness and what has caused it.

Maybe I was working out too much. Maybe overtraining in the gym taxed my adrenal glands, fried my nervous system, and weakened my immune responses, leaving me with insufficient hormone levels, intense neurological problems, and a vulnerability to pathogens like the Epstein-Barr virus. Maybe I had an undiagnosed brain or spinal cord injury from the car accident, which contributed to my illness, like how an abscessed tooth can cause meningitis. Or maybe it's something entirely unknown, something that remains undiscovered in my body. The only thing that's certain is that I've been sick for more than three years, and there's no telling how much longer this illness could last.

The possibility of being sick for the rest of my life now seems real, a feeling of existential doom. It's the sum of my fears, a deeply sad thought, and an even sadder story when it's told by people who have lived it, like the stories I've read in online forums. It's hard to imagine being sick that long. Is it really possible to have this illness for decades? I guess that's why it's called a chronic illness. But damn, I didn't know chronic meant permanent. What would it even feel like to be sick that long? What would it do to my outlook on life? I hope I don't find out. I must believe that my health will return, that the fatigue will become strength and energy, that the nausea will disappear, if not for a hangover or bad burrito, and that I'll get back to lifting weights and teaching group fitness classes.

Being well again will give me the chance to redo parts of my life—the workouts, the romances, the aspirations—but healthier and smarter. I'll teach my group fitness classes and be a better trainer. I won't judge my clients by how often they make it to class, or whether they succeed in transforming their bodies. I'll tell them to be happy with the effort they put in and not to think about anyone else's expectations. I'll encourage them to focus on how they feel, rather than how other people think they should look. And I'll apply the same idea to my own training.

I'll start lifting weights again, but I won't care what other people think of my body; I won't care whether I take home a stupid bodybuilding trophy. I'll work out because I love it. And I'll do it safer. I won't take the synthetic supplements I used to—no more caffeine pills or pre-workout supplements that have words like "explode" or "jacked" on the packaging, no more protein powder flavored like an ice cream sundae. And no more three-hour workouts. If I get carried away and work out too much, I'll rest and let my body recover before I put it through more stress, because rest days, weeks, even months, are just as important as the actual exercise. It will be a better approach than I had before. It will add longevity to the thing I love most in this world—working out—the thing I've missed so greatly and have dreamed about so vividly while I've been sick.

Working out won't be the only thing I will experience again. One day I'll randomly ask out a pretty woman at the gym. We will grow to love each other, dismissing our shortcomings and peccadilloes. She will be the first woman I truly love romantically. Sometimes we will go to concerts and bars, but more often, we will prefer to stay in and watch old movies. We will be happy and healthy together. We will get married—an intimate ceremony at an old church in San Francisco—and have two children. I'll be the best father and husband I can be. Together, the four of us, will create our own little world filled with love and fun and a sense that everything, at least for the time being, is perfect.

This recovery of mine will not be spontaneous, but when it happens—and it *will* happen—there are things I'll be inspired to do, things that I previously missed out on because I was too busy working out in the gym, too focused on my macronutrient intake and the striations in my muscles. I'll be like a prison inmate smelling fresh air again, breaking the shackles and running free. I will step out into the big, broad, beautiful world and, as the sun hits my face, I will enjoy people and places and things like I never have before.

My renewed health will be a prized possession, and I will honor it by seizing as many moments as I can, doing things I would've never done before my illness.

I will go on adventures—riding the Univega down the length of the California coast, hiking up Half Dome in Yosemite, and summiting Mount Whitney, the highest peak in the contiguous United States. But my grandest adventure will be on the water. Over several days, I will kayak down the Sacramento River, through the San Joaquin Delta and Carquinez Strait, then finally sail into the San Francisco Bay and around the Golden Gate Bridge. On the way back, paddling down the Carquinez Strait, I'll catch a glimpse of the Napa River Bridge, tempting me to take a detour and, for the first time, return to the scene of the car accident. But as the sun sets behind me, I'll decide to postpone the symbolic moment.

Then, a few days later, I will get in my car, fill up with gas just off Highway 4 in Martinez, drive up Cummings Skyway and descend, or more like float, down to Highway 37 and on to the Napa River Bridge. I will drive up the incline, holding my breath as I approach the part of the bridge where my life changed forever, where my force met fate. I will pull over to the shoulder, put my hazard lights on, and step out of the car onto the blemished concrete. I will walk to the edge of the bridge, grip the railing, and stare down at the placid water. Then I will look up at the calm sky. There will be no clouds, no wind hitting my face like thumbtacks. I will take a deep breath and inspect the concrete shoulder. There will be no flames, no thick plume of black smoke wafting through the sky, no deluge of gasoline running down the bridge. Behind me there will be no line of cars backed up on the highway, no firefighters or paramedics, and best of all, there will be no loss of life—quite the opposite, in fact.

YEAR 4

Free Fall

CHAPTER 38

Confusion Rather than Condescension

March 22, 2014

I've returned to Santa Cruz after staying with my mom for a couple of months, but I have yet to get back to my baseline level of health, which is why two filmmakers, Ryan Prior and Nicole Castillo, are coming to my studio to film me today. They're making a documentary about patients with chronic fatigue syndrome called *Forgotten Plague*. They interviewed me last July and thought a follow-up interview in my current condition would add more context to my part in the film.

I'm asleep when they arrive at the glass door to my studio. They knock and wake me up, then I open the door and welcome them inside. As soon as I shut the door, I lie back down because standing makes me dizzy and is a struggle for my weakened muscles.

Ryan makes tea for us while Nicole sets up the lighting and camera equipment before we start the interview. Like me, Ryan was an athlete who suddenly got sick and was subsequently diagnosed with chronic fatigue syndrome. He tells me that they just finished filming someone named Whitney Dafoe, who is bedridden and so profoundly ill that he has to get most of his nutrition intravenously. Ryan shows me a photo of the gaunt man in a dark room with an IV pole nearby. I don't doubt that Whitney and I have the same illness, but being that sick is hard to fathom, like trying to imagine what life would be like on another planet. I'm sick but I can still feed myself, take a shower, talk on the phone, and watch TV. Whitney can do none of those things.

Even so, he is by no means the first person to be severely sick with this illness. Sophia Mirza, a young woman from the UK, was bedridden for years. She endured medical neglect and abuse from authorities before she became too weak to eat or drink water, and the disease finally killed her in 2005. She was thirty-two.

Oddly, Mirza's death hasn't set off any alarms—no government agencies have investigated patients severely ill with CFS, most don't even devote much research funding to it, which is something that Ryan has been trying to change through his advocacy work.

As I talk to Ryan, he clarifies a lot of my confusion about the name of the disease. He tells me that it's called myalgic encephalomyelitis by patients in other countries, and the name is slowly catching on in the United States, which is why I've seen it called both names. Some patients call it ME/CFS as a way of abbreviating the two names together. The combined abbreviation is preferred by patients because calling it just chronic fatigue syndrome is dismissive of a bevy of symptoms beyond fatigue, and calling it myalgic encephalomyelitis may too turn out to be an inaccurate name; it may prove to describe a similar but different disease.

Ryan tells me that a lot of patients don't like either name. They think chronic fatigue syndrome sounds patronizing and leads people to delegitimize their symptoms. The contentious politics surrounding the illness and its name started in 1985 with an outbreak in Lake Tahoe. The Centers for Disease Control investigated the outbreak for nearly a month, but the physicians in charge of the investigation were skeptical of the legitimacy of the illness. They thought the patients were exaggerating their symptoms, even though there was obvious evidence that the patients were suffering from a legitimate illness—they had abnormally high Epstein-Barr antibodies, which prompted the CDC to initially call the illness chronic Epstein-Barr virus. Two years later, however, it was stamped with the name chronic fatigue syndrome and patients have hated it ever since.

It is a horrible name, one that has undoubtedly influenced how the general public sees the severity of the illness. Many people have as much sympathy for someone with a stubbed toe as they do for a person with chronic fatigue syndrome. If I have to be as sick as I am, I at least want people to take my illness seriously. I don't want a sickness that people think is voluntary, caused by too much work or too little sleep. I don't want to be stuck with chronic fatigue syndrome, a name that reflects the same skepticism the original CDC investigators had. I want people to see the illness for the havoc it's wreaked on my life. That's why I avoid using the name chronic fatigue syndrome whenever I can. On the rare occasion that I do tell someone about my illness, I often just say that I have a bad case of mono. It doesn't sound much better, but it usually elicits confusion rather than condescension, which is what I prefer.

It's not your job to explain your illness to people. You're not a doctor and you sure as shit didn't give it that joke of a name.

Nicole starts filming while Ryan and I drink tea and continue to talk about the politics of ME/CFS. Ryan explains that medical schools are particularly neglectful of the illness. He says that only twenty-eight percent of medical schools teach students about ME/CFS, and those that do offer little information, partly because there aren't many relevant clinical studies—only fifteen percent of universities do research on the illness.

Ryan also tells me that ME/CFS afflicts women at staggeringly higher rates than men, as much as four times as many by some estimates, which explains why he is one of only a few men I've come across with the illness. Ryan goes on to say that the disproportionate number of women with ME/CFS, particularly women of color, face more neglect and medical abuse from doctors than men, the thought of which is infuriating. Why do doctors and the medical establishment as a whole treat patients, especially women, so poorly?

Now I can see why Ryan is passionate about advocating for doctors and people in general to take this illness seriously. His advocacy is inspiring and makes me want to get more involved in the ME/CFS community. I'm passionate about the cause, but I struggle with my insecurities about living with a chronic illness. In some ways I'm still in denial about being sick. I would rather cling to my old life of throwing weights around the gym than accept the reality of the debilitated life I currently live.

The interview continues into the night, and Nicole turns on another bright light that zaps what little cognitive energy I have left. We keep filming though, and I eventually make it through the interview. Then Nicole turns off the lights, and Ryan helps her pack up the equipment and we say goodbye.

I enjoyed the visit. It was nice to spend time with people my age who understand the perils of what I'm going through. I hope their documentary finally sheds some light on this illness and the patients who have it.

CHAPTER 39

———

I Won't Allow It

November 22, 2014

The sunlight streams past the spiderwebs and raccoon droppings on top of the skylight in my studio and straight into my burning eyes. The sun seems brighter than it usually is, or maybe I've become more sensitive to it.

I lie down on my futon and throw a blanket over my head and close my eyes. It's hard not to think about how the life I've created is once again slipping from my grasp. It seems that there's nothing I can do to stop it. I've noticed my health steadily declining over the past few months, but around Halloween it really started to get bad. And now I'm too weak and in too much pain to stand for more than a couple minutes. Walking anywhere on my own is nearly impossible. It feels like I'm in the midst of a full relapse of this illness, as if it restarted itself worse than it's ever been.

Rita has been nice enough to make me meals, and my dad often brings me groceries, but now that my condition has gotten so bad, my mom is taking me back to Tuolumne so she can care for me. This comes after my latest lab results—ordered by a new doctor named Resneck-Sannes—revealed the Epstein–Barr virus has reactivated in my body. Coincidentally, Dr. Resneck-Sannes was the first physician to give me a checkup when I was an infant. Perhaps that's why I have an unusual amount of faith in him, especially given my unsuccessful history with doctors.

Another reason for my worsening condition could be that I've been using what little energy I have to work full-time from home as an editorial assistant, which I now realize is idiotic given how sick I am. Lately I spend between twenty and twenty-three hours a day in bed, a disproportionate amount of which I work on my laptop. Some days I can't even make myself a meal because I feel so sick and use all my energy to work. It's a cruel existence, a vicious cycle of illness and work exhaustion, so I've decided to cut back. Last week I told my boss that I was reducing my work hours. He wasn't happy about it. And while I should be more concerned with my health, it's hard not to think about work when I need the income.

I'm still lying on the futon when my phone buzzes beside me. My boss is calling, which he usually does at least once a day. I ignore the call and then hear a knock on the front door. My mom opens it and walks in. There's a sad, worried look on her face as she sits on the futon next to me.

"How are you, sweetie?" she asks.

"Not good. My boss just called. I don't know what to tell him."

"Just say that you're sick. You can always work when you're feeling better."

"But I'll lose my job if I can't work."

"That's okay. There will be other jobs," she says. "Try not to worry about it for now. Try not to worry about anything, okay?" I nod reluctantly as my mom rubs my back. "I'm going to pack your stuff so when the time comes you just need to get in the car."

I try to rest, but it's hard—everything in my life feels at best uncertain and at worst deteriorating. My mom finishes gathering my things, then there's another knock at the door. It's Stanley. My mom has asked him to help carry me to the car. But I won't allow it. I won't let anyone carry me.

My legs shake uncontrollably as I lift myself off the futon and try to stand up. Then suddenly my feet slip on the tiled floor, and I lose my balance and start to fall over. Stanley quickly throws my right arm over his shoulder and my mom does the same with my left arm. Together they support my weight as I hobble to the front door. I feel so weak, so fragile, so embarrassed by my body. I push the feelings aside and make it out of my studio, where the air is fresh and moist. My feet shuffle toward the driveway while I soak up the last sea breeze I may get for a while.

Walking to the car is a struggle. I have to stop and rest several times while my mom and Stanley patiently support my body weight. I finally make it to the car and Stanley opens the door for me. I hold his arm as I get in the backseat and lie down. Then he closes the door and talks with my mom.

"Kathleen, do you think it's just depression from his car accident?" Stanley asks.

Oh, not this shit again. Why does everyone think your illness is "just depression?" Stanley's like all the other people who blame this disease on being depressed. He just carried you, a grown ass man, to the car because your legs gave out and you couldn't walk, and he thinks that's depression? People like him who correlate the car accident and depression with your illness don't know shit. They just don't. The accident was traumatic; there's no argument there. But this illness is physical. It wasn't caused by mental trauma. How could even the worst psychological trauma and depression cause such prolonged and severe physical debilitation?

If Stanley and all the people who diminish your illness think you only suffer from depression, they must also think that your worst physical symptoms aren't real. It's like they think you're a big faker—a human leech orchestrating this giant ruse to get sympathy and favors for being sick, as if it's the only way you will feel fulfilled in this life. Do they think you hate doing things on your own? Do they think you don't like making food for yourself and walking without help? Even if that were somehow true, the dedication involved would be too intricate for you. It would be an Oscar-worthy performance, and you're not a good actor. You would have to be absolutely deranged to put on such a charade, to fake having to crawl to the bathroom and sit in the shower when no one is around, to wear earplugs and sunglasses while watching a movie because the sensory stimulation is too much. Of all the self-conscious people in the world, you would not have your daily life become so laughable unless it was entirely out of your control. You would have to want to be sick more than anything in the bountiful, perk-filled world.

I try to forget about Stanley's ignorant question, but there are so many things I want to say to him, and everyone else who has been skeptical of my illness. I want to tell them that depression is a serious condition, but it's a different mechanism than what is causing my illness. My body is in excruciating pain almost all the time, I constantly feel like vomiting, and I'm so weak I can't even walk to the damn car on my own. That's not depression, that's something attacking my body, something more sophisticated than even most doctors seem to understand. Whatever is the cause of my illness, it's a mistake to call it "just depression," both because depression is serious and because ME/CFS is an entirely different condition. To do so is not only wrong and confusing to patients with ME/CFS, but it marginalizes people with depression.

No illness, physical or mental, should be preceded by the word *just*. Calling a physical illness "just depression" is the kind of ignorance that stigmatizes depressed people, and in turn, lumps patients with chronic illnesses like ME/CFS into that same group of people whose suffering is wrongly deemed insignificant and unimportant by much of society.

These are the thoughts that stew in my mind as my mom drives off with me lying down in the back of the car. I do my best to shut off my brain, and to forget about all the bad stuff happening inside my body.

YEAR 5

Bedridden

CHAPTER 40

No ER

January 25 – 26, 2015

On top of the Epstein–Barr virus reactivating in my body, I now have the flu, which my mom brought home from work last week. I specifically remember saying I wouldn't catch it, but I must have jinxed myself because two days ago it hit me hard with a fever and nasal congestion. The congestion has made it difficult for me to sleep, so tonight I'm taking a generic cold medicine that will hopefully help.

A few hours after drinking the cough syrup, I wake up in a cold sweat and go to the bathroom. My heart races as I try to pee standing up, then my legs tremble and give out, and I collapse on the toilet. I'm too weak to stand up, so I just sit there and pee while the light above the sink rattles my brain. It burns my eyes, rendering me motionless. I rest my head in my hands while short, heavy breaths explode from my chest.

When I've regained enough strength, I get back on my feet and stumble to my mom's bedroom, but the door is shut, so I return to bed as intense weakness consumes my body. I don't know if I'll be able to get up again. It seems the Epstein–Barr virus, flu, and cold medicine have done me in.

I reach for the phone next to my pillow and send my mom a text message. She wakes up and comes to my room.

"Mom, I'm not doing well. My heart is racing, and I'm really weak."

"Oh, sweetie, I'm sorry." She scans my face. "You don't look good. Should we go to the ER?"

"No. They won't understand."

"I know," she says. "But I'm worried."

My mom calls an advice nurse, but because I'm no longer on her health insurance, the woman won't help, except to advise that I go to the hospital. After I insist she not take me to the ER, my mom lies at the foot of my bed and falls asleep while I continue fighting the symptoms throughout the night.

* * *

It's morning and I wake up with my mom still asleep in my bed. I'm even weaker than last night. The level of sickness I feel is hard to express, except to say that it's the worst I've ever felt. I'm extremely weak, breathing is difficult, and talking is nearly impossible. Moving my body is so strenuous that I can't even lift my arms and legs off the mattress. And my eyes have become so sensitive to light that I must keep them covered. Sound is also hard to tolerate, even ambient noises—doors closing, microwaves beeping, water running—it's all amplified, like an air horn blaring in my ears.

This is the stuff of nightmares—I'm trapped in my own body, and I don't know if I have the strength to ask for help. When I try to speak, my mom doesn't hear the faint whisper.

When I click my tongue against the roof of my mouth, she still doesn't respond. Finally I roll over and bump my mom to get her attention.

"Do you need something?" she asks, rising groggily from the foot of the bed.

"Help," I whisper.

"Oh, kiddo." My mom looks at me with a panicked expression. I don't know what she sees, but it must be upsetting because tears are falling down her face. "I'm calling an ambulance. We're going to the ER," she insists. My mom digs around the bed for her phone, nervous energy shooting out of her and bouncing around the room as she tries to save her sick son from the illness ravaging his body.

"No," I say.

"Yes, we're going to the emergency room."

"No ER." I force out the words. Saying more than one word is incredibly difficult, like trying to talk underwater with my mouth closed.

"Fine, then I'm going to call the doctor."

My mom reaches Dr. Resneck-Sannes on his cell phone. He's unique in his attentiveness—the only doctor I've known to take phone calls away from the office, which only adds to my appreciation of him. He spent an hour with me during my last visit, and now he's on the phone with my mom before his office is even open, looking over my recent lab results. Realizing the urgency of the situation, the doctor quickly calls in a prescription for an antiviral medication.

My mom drives to the pharmacy and returns with the medication, then I swallow a pill the size of a Tootsie Roll, which I'm supposed to take three times a day. Within the hour, I no longer feel on the precipice of death. I don't know if the antiviral is working, but for now my fever is gone and my condition is stable.

CHAPTER 41

It Won't Be Forever

February 10, 2015

My mom is seated beside my bed. I look at her, then pinch my thumb and index finger together in front of my lips as if I'm sucking from a straw.

"A joint? You want a joint?" my mom asks with confusion and a hint of playfulness.

I try to laugh, wince, then shake my head and point to the water glass and straw sitting on the bedside table.

"Oh, water. You want water." My mom grabs the glass and holds it for me as I painfully suck water from the straw. Once I've finished drinking, she returns the glass to the bedside table.

"Are you sure you don't want a joint?" she asks.

We give each other a look and tacitly acknowledge the ridiculousness of the situation, the absurdity of what we've been going through. The glass of water I just drank from is the closest I've come to running water since I last got out of bed two weeks ago. Since then, I haven't been able to brush my teeth, use the toilet, or bathe. Though yesterday I did desperately try to get to the bathroom, only to fail miserably.

Because I can't walk, or even stand up, the plan was for me to lie down on a snowboard (yes, a snowboard), and have my mom push me across the floor until I reached the bathroom. But when the time came, my body wouldn't cooperate. I gingerly sat up and slid off the bed onto the snowboard and curled up in a fetal position. But as my mom pushed me across the carpeted floor, I became too sick to continue and eventually retreated to bed, where I've remained mostly motionless for the last day or so. The thought of my mom pushing a one hundred and sixty-pound man across the floor on a snowboard was amusing, but the pain I felt wasn't. If she had kept going, it would have only made me sicker.

The first twelve hours after my snowboard excursion was the worst. My body filled with intense pain and weakness so profound that I could barely move. Then my body flared with a tantrum of other symptoms—the fever returned, and my heart rate reached upward of one hundred and seventy beats per minute, which would be fine for someone on a jog, but not a sick person lying flat and motionless in bed. In contrast, the last time I tried to do a few push-ups, more than a year ago, my heart rate was barely above one hundred.

Now, as I lie in bed trying to sip water from a straw, my heart rate has steadied, but there's a new problem: communication. I've lost my ability to speak. Sometimes I can whisper a few words, but never loudly enough for my mom to hear. A couple weeks ago I was speaking thousands of words a day; now I'm stuck futilely whispering only a few.

Thankfully, I'm able to translate most of my needs using hand signals. I point to my stomach for food and pretend to smoke a joint if I need water. When nature calls, I either use a water bottle that my mom has affectionately deemed "the pee bottle," or for a bowel movement, I show her two fingers and she brings in a bucket that I squat on next to the bed. It's not the weightlifting squats of my past, but somehow it's even more taxing on my muscles. I was so embarrassed the first time I slid the bucket back to my mom, but in her comforting way she assured me that "It's just like this now. It won't be forever."

I can't help but notice the similarities between how I felt when I first got sick with mono in 2010 and this latest relapse. The difference now is that my condition is significantly worse. When I initially had mono, I could still speak and get out of bed to go to the bathroom. Now I can't. But I'm still holding on to the hope that soon this stage of the illness will improve, and I can get back to my life in Santa Cruz.

It seems, for the moment, that some energy has returned to my body. I should savor this little bit of relief from my symptoms, but after hours of doing nothing, my mind wants to do something. I'm tired of the boredom, pain, and fatigue. I want excitement, passion, and pleasure. I want to escape this hell I'm in, so I grab my phone and search a few explicit keywords. Within seconds I'm watching a video of two people having sex, if you can even call it that. It's sloppy and unromantic—two strangers objectifying their bodies so I can live vicariously through them. I can't stop watching, but my body isn't doing well. The stimulation is too much for me to handle. The worst symptoms are back—my head is pounding, and my heart is racing as weakness consumes my muscles. Perhaps I too have objectified my body. Everything hurts. I have no choice but to turn my phone off and hide it under my bed so I don't do further damage to my health.

CHAPTER 42

A Step Above a Corpse

March 11, 2015

I've been bedridden for the past six weeks, leaving me with a constant fear that death will swallow me up at any moment. As frightening as the feeling is, it has forced me to surrender to the mercy of this illness. In that way, it has been simpler for me to let go of my obligations, though I can feel my fear and resentment about it being bottled up inside me, waiting to be released at a later, healthier time. Until then, I have to accept the fact that I don't have the strength or energy to properly grieve the parts of my life that I've lost.

Thankfully my mom has made it as easy as possible by handling most of my affairs. She called Rita and Stanley and told them I couldn't pay rent on my studio anymore and that my dad would need to move my stuff out. Then, when my boss called for the fifth time in one day, my mom answered and stepped out of the room to talk to him. I heard her say, "He can't talk. He's too sick."

There are many more things my mom will have to settle for me in the coming weeks—credit card and student loan payments, unanswered emails—so many things, in fact, that I've had to grant her power of attorney. The hard part wasn't trusting my mom with the responsibility, nor was it relinquishing control of my affairs; it was writing my name on the stupid documents. I didn't even have the strength to hold the damn pen.

I'm still plagued by that weakness. I feel it in every part of my body, every muscle fiber and bone. I feel it in my fingers and hands when I pinch the straw in my water glass. I even feel it in my mouth and jaw when I sip from the straw. The weakness is so profound that, when I try to eat food, my mouth just won't work. I can't move my jaw enough to chew anything. I feel the weakness in every tiny muscle of my face. But it doesn't stop there. I feel it in my toes, even in my eyes. When it's really bad, my vision starts to flicker like a home movie from the sixties. It's all so degrading. But, despite it all, my brain still works reasonably well. My mind is vivid and alive, even though my body is barely a step above a corpse.

I might as well be in a coma. Life would certainly be easier—I wouldn't need to turn on my side and defecate into a garbage bag now that I'm too weak to squat on a bucket beside my bed; I wouldn't need my mom to brush my teeth every morning; I wouldn't need a plastic urinal constantly attached to my hip; and I wouldn't need to drink my meals through a straw. Although these things have made my life livable, they have also made it infinitely more pathetic.

I'm in desperate need of medical care, but because Tuolumne is in such a remote area, it's impossible to find a doctor who will make a house call. And going to the ER is pointless, probably even counterproductive. No ER doctor in rural California is going to understand an illness that a specialist like Dr. Peterson couldn't even treat effectively. Not to mention the ER would have bright lights, a cacophony of loud noises, and I'd have to take a bumpy twenty-minute ambulance ride just to get there. I'm afraid my body couldn't handle any of it.

For now I'm settling for the frequent contact my mom keeps with Dr. Resneck-Sannes in Santa Cruz. He still has me taking the antiviral medication, which so far has done little besides reduce my fever, but luckily he's been able to find a home health nurse to do a checkup and blood draw on me.

The nurse arrives and makes her way up the same stairs I ascended one at a time while sitting on my ass not three months ago. I can hear and feel her ascent, the weight of her body reverberating through the floorboards.

I wave to the middle-aged, burly woman when she enters my darkened room.

"Hi, Jamison. I'm here to draw your blood," the nurse says. "I'm gonna need the light on so I can check vitals and draw blood."

"Okay, sure," my mom says standing near my bed.

The nurse flips the light on. It burns my eyes, so I cover them with an eye mask, sheet, and blanket. It feels like I'm at the bottom of a pile of coats at a party. It's hot and hard to breathe under all the layers, but it's better than facing the effects of the light in the room.

The nurse sits next to me, and I feel her slip an oxygen sensor onto my index finger.

"Your blood oxygen level is ninety-seven," she says. "That's better than mine, so you probably don't need to worry about blood clots."

The nurse proceeds to check my vitals, then forcefully grabs my arm and pulls it laterally until it hangs off the bed. Pain shoots through my arm and shoulder, then my entire body. It's intense and draining, but I need to get this checkup done. The blood work is my best shot at understanding the cause of my relapse. So I let the nurse have her way with me, but any comfort I felt knowing I'm under medical care has now vanished. I just want this all to be over.

The nurse doesn't ease up. She yanks my arm farther off the bed, then pushes down on my forearm so the blood flow will increase. My elbow is on top of the mattress and my forearm pushed below the bed frame. It hurts so much it feels like I may pass out and, because I can't speak, neither my mom nor the nurse knows I'm in pain. It's a stark contrast to the last time I had my blood drawn five months ago. The nurse was gentler then, but also, I must be more sensitive to pain now. Getting my blood drawn shouldn't hurt this much, no matter how rough the nurse is. It feels like I've become this fragile thing, a delicate human made of glass.

"I'm just trying to find a good vein. I always find one," the nurse says.

Suddenly I feel a sharp jab to the inside of my elbow. At first, I think it's the needle going into my arm, but then I feel another jab hit the same spot. I can't see what the nurse is doing, but I think she's hitting my arm with her fist. It hurts like hell.

"Just a couple more taps and I should have a vein," the nurse says.

Taps? This lady is throwing haymakers on your arm, and she thinks they're taps.

I can feel the nurse's warm skin against mine and the rush of air made by her "taps." Each time she hits my arm, she makes an aggressive guttural sound. It gives me a primal reaction, like I'm wrestling someone, except I can't wrestle. I can barely even move.

The pain is so bad I want to cry out for help, but it's no use. I can't even whisper. So I just suck it up. I take it all—the pain and humiliation, the nausea and wanting to vomit, the utter weakness and exhaustion.

I may be wrong, but I honestly believe this is a necessary, beneficial step in my healing.

CHAPTER 43

Protein

April 22, 2015

The results from the latest blood draw ordered by Dr. Resneck-Sannes have come back, and my mom has been spending lots of time on the phone with him discussing potential treatment options. This is time beyond the doctor's regular office hours, time that he's not charging me for. In this way Dr. Resneck-Sannes is quite a contrast to Dr. Peterson, whom my mom also recently called for advice about my relapse. The receptionist at his office told my mom to write up a summary of my condition, just like I did three years ago before my first appointment with Dr. Peterson. My mom went through the agony of reliving everything that has happened in the last few months, then faxed the summary to the doctor. She waited weeks for a response, and when someone from Dr. Peterson's office finally called her, it was an oblivious intern who said the doctor wouldn't be able to help me. He couldn't even spare five minutes to answer a simple question.

Now the only glimmer of hope I have is Dr. Resneck-Sannes. The blood tests he ordered showed that I'm malnourished, deficient in several key nutrients, especially protein. It has been extremely difficult for me to get any substantial source of protein through a straw, which is still the only way I can consume food. Luckily as a former bodybuilder, I'm good at finding creative ways of getting protein. Right now that means drinking more protein shakes than I drank when I was bodybuilding. The problem is that too much concentrated protein powder will inevitably make someone constipated. Today that someone is me. I haven't taken a shit in six days, and I'm starting to worry. It's quite painful. And needing my mom's help doesn't make it any easier.

She's sitting beside my bed. I motion for her to come closer, then I take her hand and trace the word *clogged* on it with my finger. I would have traced *constipated*, but it has too many letters.

"What's clogged?" my mom asks. I point to myself. "You're clogged?"

I nod and show her two fingers, the hand signal I use for when I need a bowel movement.

"Oh, I see," she says. "Well, you can try a laxative, but things might get messy. The only other option I can think of is a suppository."

Well, doesn't that sound fun?

It's not easy weighing the discomfort of constipation against that of having an object shoved up my ass. But, ultimately, I decide to do it.

An hour after what I fully expect to be the most uncomfortable moment I will ever share with my mom, I again show her two fingers. Then I roll on my side as she slides an absorbent pad and garbage bag under my hip. It feels good to relieve myself, but shame soon follows as my mom enters the room with baby wipes and a wet washcloth to clean me up, a lengthy process that I prefer to do in the dark with my eyes closed. I try not to think about the humiliation of needing my mother to help me clean myself, but it's impossible not to focus on.

Five years ago I was living on my own, working out every day with a giant tractor tire, about to graduate college; now I can't even wipe my own ass. I don't know how I got here, how my life degenerated to this point. It absolutely blows my mind that this has become my reality, that my new existence has been widdled down to lying in bed, trying to survive, and not shit myself. It's almost comical, except it's not.

CHAPTER 44

Swamp

May 7, 2015

I'm in a square room, lying on a rectangular twin mattress, the third I've gone through in recent months. Since I've been bed-ridden, I have become a destroyer of mattresses. I've managed to spill every liquid imaginable on them, but I prefer to blame the real damage on gravity. Because I'm too weak to get up, my mattresses have had to support my weight constantly. They never get a chance to breathe, the coils never unfold, and inevitably the mattress begins to sink in around my immobile body like a tortilla enveloping taco fillings. Then I have to move to a new bed, which, once again, I did yesterday. It was exhausting.

Since moving to the new bed, I've been trying to rest and let my body recover. The room I'm in is completely dark, and I have no idea what time it is. My best guess is it's around nine in the morning, because I can see bits of sunlight peeking through the blanket pinned over the window and blinds. Though, it could be mid-afternoon and I wouldn't know it. There's no clock in my room, and my mom has hidden my phone from me because looking at the bright screen only makes me sicker. I've also been regularly sleeping past noon, so the time of day that someone usually comes to check on me very much remains a mystery. I wouldn't care so much, but beside me on the tiny twin mattress is a plastic urinal with at least ten hours' worth of my piss in it. I cannot fill it any higher, and I feel another urge to pee coming on.

The house is quiet, no one seems to be coming to help me. Trying my hardest not to spill the liter of piss leaning against my hip, I slowly shimmy my body closer to the bedside table where there's an empty water glass. I move the glass next to my hip and fill most of it with the contents of my bladder, but as I return the glass to the table it proves too heavy for my weakened muscles. The glass slips from my fingers onto the urinal, and like a row of dominoes, both tip over, spilling on me and the mattress. It's a river of warm and cold urine flowing on and around me. If it didn't smell so bad, it might actually be refreshing; it's the closest thing to a shower that I've had in months.

My initial reaction is to panic, and I do. I panic as much as an immobile, mostly silent person can. I even make an audible sound, which is more of a whimper and much to my embarrassment sounds like a lonely dog left out in the rain—I'm the lonely dog and the rain is my urine.

Several minutes pass and I'm still soaked in piss. I want to scream for help, for this madness to stop. Nobody deserves a piss bath and being forgotten in a dark room. This is no way to live, silent and soaking in my own urine. I want it all to end. I want this life to end, but not necessarily because it's too hard or I'm suffering too much, but because there's no end to my misery in sight. It's been months without any substantial improvement to my health. I've had to accept that there may never be an improvement; this may be it. I may one day die on this urine-stained mattress.

Until then, however, I must numbly get through this cruel experience just as I've survived the many other white-knuckle moments I've been through in the last few years. I've developed an almost subconscious mechanism to deal with the countless hazards of being bedridden: urinal spills, bowel movements, or the time my mom was feeding me and spilled a container of hot French onion soup on my chest, or another time when my dad tripped and regained his balance by planting all of his weight on my fragile body. These are the unavoidable struggles of being cared for in bed.

I hear two voices bickering outside the door—a hostile and clandestine meeting about my failing health. The voices are unmistakably those of my mom and my dad, who have been switching off as my caregiver and essentially living together part-time, two decades removed from divorce, with the sole purpose of healing their son. Spending so much time together has made them combatants, which is difficult for me to witness. But right now I don't care about their disagreements; I just want them to open the door and clean the piss off me. One of the two should check on me soon, probably my dad because today is his turn to care for me before he drives back home to Santa Cruz tomorrow.

Whoever walks through the door will have their hands full, a bed and body soaked in urine and in desperate need of cleaning. Still, it won't be as bad as the bowel movements, which we're all still getting used to, especially considering that when I became bedridden, neither of my parents had seen me naked since I was a kid.

I hear my bedroom door slowly open, then my dad's bearded face peeks through a foot-sized opening. With it comes new air and a burst of morning aromas—roasted coffee and fried eggs—which mingle with the stale stench of urine before giving way to it completely. I expect my dad to come in the room, but he doesn't, so I tap on the urinal to get his attention. He starts to back away and close the door. I wave my hands at him, but he can't see me in the dark. Just as the door is about to shut, I whisper, "help," which to me feels like yelling, but to my dad must sound as unrecognizable as a faint noise outside.

When the door closes, I am enraged and despondent. I want to fight and cry at the same time. But I don't do either. I remain immobile, stewing in a swamp of piss.

CHAPTER 45

Big, Bulbous Tears

May 28, 2015

My dad is back from Santa Cruz and on caregiving duty. But things aren't going well. It's not that I'm unappreciative of my dad's help, it's that we are both impatient and my standard of living is higher than his. My dad hasn't always taken the best care of himself. For two years he lived in a tree house on top of a mountain, and not the trendy tree houses people pay three hundred dollars a night to rent on Airbnb. His tree house had no running water and was full of rat droppings and mold. That's probably why when I labored through a series of hand signals earlier tonight to ask him to replace the dirty straw in my water glass, he seemed bothered and unsympathetic.

Now he's setting up my nighttime urinal, a new invention I orchestrated, again through hand signals. It's a simple work of makeshift engineering that has significantly reduced my incidence of urine spills at night. It consists of thick tubing with a valve on one end that is placed on my bed, while the other end sits in a bucket on the floor. The tube is bungeed to a stool so I can still reach it if it falls off my bed. My dad doesn't get the importance of the bungee cord and, because he's inept at reading my hand signals, we get frustrated with each other.

"What are you trying to tell me, son?" he asks. I point to the tube for the fifth time.

"I see you pointing, but what do you want me to do?"

Attach the tube to the stool.

I point to the stool, but it seems to only intensify the perplexed look on his face. Not knowing what else to do, I again point to the stool.

"Son, I see you pointing, but I don't know what you want." I'm exasperated. I point to the tube, then the stool. "The stool? You want me to take it away?" My dad grabs the stool and carries it toward the door. Frantic and frustrated, I tap on the tube to get his attention.

"Okay, what now?" He brings the stool back and looks annoyed.

I bristle at his irritated tone, then jab my finger at the tube.

"Yes, the tube. What about it?" my dad asks.

Attach the fucking tube to the stool.

I point to the stool.

"The stool? You just told me to move it." My dad huffs, looks at me incredulously, and throws up his hands. "You're driving me fucking nuts."

My body fills with rage and I growl at him, which to me feels like I'm screaming but it's actually quite faint, even to my ears. The growl sounds worn and distant, as if I've been trapped in a bathroom at a concert, yelling for someone to rescue me. This attempt at expressing my anger is all I can muster. I can't speak and hand signals don't seem to work with my dad. It's as if I'm playing the world's worst version of charades, an all-too serious game in which the players grow increasingly hostile and angry with one another. But to me it's not a game—it's my life.

My dad looks at me, his face pained. "Son, I'm . . ." His voice catches in his throat. He tries to speak again, but sadness overtakes him, and his chest begins to heave. I can't remember ever seeing him cry, even when he had cancer and went through several rounds of chemotherapy. He was gaunt and always running to the bathroom to vomit, but I never once saw him break down and cry. Now here he is, struggling to help his sick son as big, bulbous tears well up in his eyes. The tears slide down his face, and I'm confronted by his sniffling, as compassion and regret erase my frustration and rage.

I've always known my dad to be exceptionally patient, but everyone has a limit. We both reached our limits tonight, and it's because of me. It's because I can't get up to go to the bathroom, or even speak to tell my dad what I need.

I want to hug my dad and apologize for this ridiculous situation. I want to convey my gratitude for all he has done for me. But before I can reach for his hand to express myself, he turns and walks out of the room.

I hate this so much. I would do anything to not have to be here right now, to revert to a better time, a more pleasant experience in which I can just enjoy spending time with my dad. I want to go back to my childhood when, at the height of my sports obsession, my dad and I would get up early on Saturdays and sell my baseball cards at the flea market, the smell of Coppertone lingering between us as we sat out in the sun. I miss the simplicity of that time, my little world revolving around baseball cards and spending the day outside with my dad. Now my world revolves around trying to get him to set up my overnight urinal. It feels like my worst nightmare, futilely trying to get someone I love to do something so simple and so necessary, yet so impossible without speaking.

What seems like an hour goes by before my dad returns, his head bowed. "Okay, son, I'm sorry for getting weepy," he says, standing next to my bed. He sets the urinal tube down on my mattress. "I'm just going to leave the tube here. You can use it just fine. I'll sleep in here with you. Tap on something if you need me."

My dad lies down on a futon on the other side of the room and suddenly everything is quiet. Everything but my mind. How could I get so angry with someone who's just trying to keep me alive? How could I fault my dad for not possessing exceptional deductive reasoning skills? I want to say so many things to him. But I can't. Without speaking, I don't know how to tell him how much I appreciate his help. It makes me feel angry and outraged. This illness has trampled all over my life for years now, but this time it's gone too far.

This madness has to stop. I must escape this cruel alternative universe in which I have to ask my dad for help without speaking and piss into a tube and bucket instead of an actual toilet. I can't subject myself to this shit anymore. I refuse to put up with any further indignity. But I don't have a choice. No matter how inhumane my life gets, and how fed up I feel, there's not a damn thing I can do about it. There's no customer service representative to yell at, no complaint form to fill out. I can only suck it up and watch helplessly as this illness continues to destroy my body and damage the relationships I hold dearest.

CHAPTER 46

Tough Cookie

June 6 – 12, 2015

My dad has gone home, which means my mom has been pulling double-duty—working full-time as a teacher during the day and taking care of me in the evening. Tonight she seems extra exhausted, and she's all alone caring for me until my dad comes back in a few days.

She has just finished setting up my urinal and doing the rest of my nighttime routine, a dizzying sequence of tasks including, but not limited to, brushing my teeth, washing my face, and giving me medications. In addition to the antiviral drug and supplements I've been taking, I'm considering adding an antidepressant. The last time I tried this type of medication, at the direction of Dr. Gretchen, I didn't see any benefits. But I need to try something. I can't just lie here waiting for this illness to kill me. Even if the antidepressant won't treat my illness, maybe it will improve my mental health and make this situation more bearable. That way I can at least keep my mind healthy while my body battles the illness.

The antidepressant is also supposed to improve sleep and anxiety, two things that I could use some help with. My only concern is the side effects. I've always been sensitive to medications, and the last thing I need right now is side effects making my condition worse.

"Do you want to take the antidepressant?" my mom asks, standing next to my bed.

I'm still ambivalent about taking it, so I point to my temple then to my mom, which is my way of asking her what she thinks I should do.

"What do I think?" she asks. I nod. "I think you should try it." She looks tired and impatient. She just wants to go to sleep, but I'm keeping her awake with my indecisiveness.

I point to my side, hoping it will translate as my concern about side effects.

"Your ribs, do they hurt?" my mom asks.

I give a thumbs down and again point to my side. She looks at me blankly, and I realize that she's not going to guess what I'm trying to say. I try another strategy. I grab my mom's hand and trace an *S* with my index finger.

"Was that *S*?" she asks.

I give a thumbs up and trace an *I* on her hand.

"An *P*?" my mom asks. She lets out a big yawn. She looks so tired. I should stop and let her go to bed, but I don't feel good about taking the medication without knowing the side effects.

I give a thumbs up and trace *D*.

"Was that a *B*?" my mom asks.

I give a thumbs down and trace the letter again.

"I'm still getting *B*." I shake my head. She frowns and rubs her eyes. "Is it *D*?" she asks.

I give an emphatic thumbs up and start to trace the last letter.

"Side?" she asks. I nod and take a deep breath. "Is there another word?"

I nod again and trace an *E* on her hand.

"Was that *F?*"

I give a thumbs down. My mom closes her eyes and lets out a long sigh. I trace *E* again.

"I'm still getting an *F*," she says.

I shake my head and trace the letter a third time.

Just take the stupid pill already. Does it really matter if you know the side effects? It's not going to make a difference once you take the pill. You will either have the side effects or you won't.

"Was it *T?*" my mom asks.

I throw up my hands in frustration. Now it feels like I'm playing a distorted game of *Wheel of Fortune* in which I'm a grumpy Pat Sajak. Either that or I'm playing Hangman and just used my final guess.

"You know what? I'm exhausted." My mom's voice quavers and cracks, then she starts to cry. "I'm working all day and taking care of you at night. I'm at my limit. I'm in survival mode here. I need a break. If I don't get help soon, you may have to go live in a facility."

You wouldn't last a day in a long-term care facility with all the doctors and nurses who don't know shit about your illness. You have to figure something out because she can't keep going at this pace. She's nearly sixty. She needs more help than just your dad chipping in every other week. She needs respite like you need to avoid a long-term care facility.

"I gotta go to bed," she says, irritation bubbling up on her face. "I'm going to get you the antidepressant. It should help you sleep. But if you're worried, I can just give you half the dose."

My mom empties half the capsule and hands me the anti-depressant. I hesitate for a few seconds with the pill in my hand.

"What's your reluctance?" my mom asks. "I need to get to sleep, so you have to make a decision here." She pauses for a second and grabs the literature that came with the prescription. "If you're worried about a bad reaction, I'll read the side effects to you."

I can't help but smile at the absurdity—I just spent half an hour futilely trying to ask my mom to read the side effects, and now she surprisingly thought to do it on her own.

"Weakness, fatigue, vivid dreams, and a rapid heart rate."

The side effects don't sound good, but it's hard to imagine the medication making me worse than I already feel.

"Oh, just take the pill," my mom says. "You need to sleep. I need to sleep."

My mom is right. She needs a break and I need relief from my symptoms—an escape from the horrors of my circumstances. Sleep is my best shot. I pop the pill in my mouth, swallow it with water, and then close my eyes and let a dream fade in.

* * *

Somehow the sunlight shines through the blinds, past the black blanket on the window, and into my eye mask. It wakes me up in a daze, and I feel worse than before I took the antidepressant last night. My head won't stop spinning, even though my body is completely horizontal. But the weakness is the most debilitating. I can barely move, and it seems that every time I try, my heart rate soars to dangerous levels. Then the tremors start. It's as if my body won't allow me to do anything, but it has no problem shaking uncontrollably just to torment me. It doesn't make any sense. None of this does.

Terror, pure unadulterated terror, consumes me. I fear that the tremors are making my heart beat even faster, and that moving, even just to the other side of my twin bed, might be too much exertion and cause my heart to stop. It's all because of that stupid antidepressant. Weakness and a rapid heart rate were listed as the side effects. I shouldn't have taken the antidepressant. It wasn't worth it. Now all I want is for the side effects to stop, and for my health to stabilize.

* * *

It's now the middle of the night, a full day has gone by since I took the antidepressant, and my heart is still racing. I've been trying to distract myself from the side effects and the fear of what a sleepless night will do to my weakened body. I've been lying as still as possible, trying not to accelerate my heart rate. I'm afraid this illness is too strong, too aggressive for my sick body, and it's finally going to kill me. My heart is beating so fast that it could stop at any moment. But maybe that's just wishful thinking. My quality of life is so poor that I might as well be dead. There's no enjoyment in this life of misery. I can't speak or eat. I can't even move without my heart feeling like it's going to explode.

A few hours pass and I'm still fighting for my life, fighting for everything that I hold sacred—my family and friends, endless ocean views, granola on foggy mornings, Humphrey Bogart movies late at night, and a thousand other things that I miss so much.

My mom walks in to check on me, but I'm too weak to tell her how sick I am, too weak to tell her anything at all. It's just one of the many small paradoxes that make up the larger paradox that is this illness. Through an arduous sequence of faint whispers and hand gestures, I'm able to tell my mom that my pulse is racing. She hooks me up to a heart rate monitor. It shows 183 beats a minute, a scary number for someone lying flat in bed.

"I'm calling the ambulance," my mom says.

I shake my head and point to Dr. Resneck-Sannes's name printed on a pill bottle beside my bed.

"You want me to call him?" my mom asks. I weakly nod my head. "Jamison, the doctor can't do anything for you. He tried but can't help you anymore. You need to try to relax. I'm going to give you another antidepressant."

I give a thumbs down.

"Why not?" she asks. I can't tell my mom that the antidepressant is the reason my heart is racing, so I just give her another thumbs down.

"Well, you know what? That makes no sense to me. I think it's a careless decision."

Her response fills me with anger. It's not a careless decision; it's the right decision. I'm defensive but can't speak, so I let out a low growl. My message gets across—maybe it's the growl, the red in my eyes, or the tension in my body, but something makes my mom recoil.

"That's it. I'm done. I don't deserve this," she yells. I cup my ears. Her face is flushed and covered in tears. "Jamison! I . . . I don't know what else to say." She turns away and storms out of the room.

Then, before I know it, I hear the front door slam shut, and my mom's footsteps stomp down the driveway. She's gone. Everyone has a breaking point, and my mom just reached hers. She's broken. I broke her. I know she wants to save me from the grips of this illness, but maybe she can't. Maybe she's done all she can. Maybe that's why she left—she couldn't bear to fight a losing battle anymore.

It's an eerie feeling without her here. I'm all alone, unable to care for myself, and my heart continues to pound in my chest. All I can do is surrender to what is happening. I've spent so much time, so much energy, fighting this illness and desperately trying to overcome the setbacks it has caused in my life, but I've failed to see how powerless I've been. I've gotten so wrapped up in trying to control every aspect of my life that I didn't realize that my fate has been out of my hands the entire time.

I take a gulp of air and feel a warming sensation as my breath pushes back up from my lungs and out of my mouth. I take another breath and close my eyes. I'm ready to let go. Whatever happens, happens. If my heart gives out, it gives out. If I die, I die. But before I go, if that is my fate, I hope my mom knows how incredibly sorry I am that this whole ordeal has happened. I'm sorry for subjecting her to the appointments with doctors, the late nights holding my hand as I wait for my symptoms to calm down, the countless days she's had to both work and take care of me. I'm sorry that this illness has robbed us of enjoyable time together. I hate that it has tainted our bond.

Now, more than ever, I wish my mom was here. I wish she would stay with me. I wish she could just be my mom, not a caregiver keeping me alive or a surrogate searching for a doctor who knows how to treat this illness. I just want to relax and enjoy each other's company, as we used to before I got sick.

But I don't blame her for leaving. I can't imagine what it's like to see your child so sick, so weak and frail and on the precipice of death. I would probably leave, too, and run far, far away. I just hope she knows how appreciative I am that she stuck with me this long.

* * *

I'm still alive. Barely. Another full day has gone by, and I'm relieved to find that, after taking some Ativan and remaining supine for the last seventy-two hours, my pulse has slowed down. But I have a new problem: it's painful for me to pee.

It may be caused by a urinary tract infection, so I'm drinking pure cranberry juice as a remedy. I wish I could say it tastes good, but it doesn't. It's the sourest thing I've ever had, and drinking it through a straw makes me pucker even more.

While I wait for the cranberry juice to kick in, my mom walks into my room. After she stormed out of the house yesterday, she eventually came back and gave me a hug. I could tell she was too exhausted to talk about what she was feeling, or maybe she just didn't want to—maybe she thought it was pointless. And maybe she was right. In that moment, there was nothing we could do. We just had to stay there in my room, listening to each other breathe, waiting for time to pass, hoping that things got better.

Eventually we carried on and before long, my mom was back in action, taking care of me like the selfless mother she is.

Now she's standing beside my bed, holding some mail for me.

"Your friend Sasha sent you a card. Want me to read it?" my mom asks. I nod. She shows me a card with a partially eaten cookie on the front. "It says, 'Tough Cookie.'"

My mom has been talking to Sasha, who recently found out about my condition online. She told my mom she wants to come visit soon. I still have feelings for Sasha, but in my weakened state, even a friendly visit from her would be nice.

My mom puts the card beside my bed. Then she starts my hygiene routine by brushing my teeth. I've never liked going to the dentist, and my mom brushing my teeth feels almost exactly like getting a dental cleaning: a masked person jams a toothbrush in my mouth while I try my best not to choke or swallow the toothpaste. My mom does this daily, while wearing a mask so I don't catch another virus.

After I rinse my mouth and spit into a bucket, we move on to a sponge bath. First, my mom covers my bed in absorbent pads, then rubs soap on me, then rinses it off with a spray bottle and a washcloth. I can feel my mom's pent-up anger and grief as she rubs a sudsy cloth across my torso. The pressure from her hands inflames my muscles and ignites a fight or flight response within me. Each stroke of the cloth feels like she's washing me with a heavy rock in her hand.

I try to wash myself as much as possible, especially in my private areas, but it's incredibly draining and makes my heart beat faster, so I have to stop and take lots of breaks. In all, the sponge bath takes an hour or two and does the same thing many people can accomplish with a five-minute shower. Because it's so painful and exhausting, most days the sponge bath includes just the dirtiest areas of my body, or what I think of as *pits, tits,* and *bits.*

My mom giving me sponge baths is awkward, but it's not the most uncomfortable moment we've had, and it's definitely better than not washing off the sweat and other bodily fluids that accumulate on my skin every day.

That's to say, as bad as all of this is, it could be worse. It could always be worse.

* * *

The cranberry juice didn't work, and now I can't pee at all. It constantly feels like I have to relieve myself but I can't, and by the looks of the large bulge forming just below my belly button, my bladder is retaining the fluids I've been drinking.

My mom notices I haven't been peeing, and her maternal instinct kicks in. She takes my temperature, something I never would have thought to do. The thermometer shows 101.3 degrees.

"You could have something serious going on," my mom says. "If you can't pee, I'm sorry, but we have to go to the ER." I groan and let out a long sigh. "You'll be okay. I'm going to be there with you to make sure of it."

My mom is right—this could be serious. The ER doctors probably won't know how to treat ME/CFS, but hopefully they can solve my bladder problem. I give my mom a thumbs up, and she calls an ambulance. Then I prepare for the chaos to come. I wear earplugs, an eye mask, and sunglasses to protect my senses and keep my symptoms from flaring up at the hospital. I probably look odd with all the stuff on my head, but I'm far beyond caring what I look like at this point. If there's one good thing that's come from being this sick, it's that the vanity I used to have when I was a bodybuilder now seems frivolous and immature. I'm too concerned with surviving to care about how I look.

A few minutes later I'm surrounded by a group of first responders, all trying to strategize how to transport me downstairs and into the ambulance. I peek from underneath my eye mask and sunglasses and see two male firefighters, two male EMTs, and a female paramedic.

Do they really need all these people to carry you? In your condition, you probably weigh as much as a child.

I hear someone say, "You're up, Diane."

Then a soft female voice beside me says: "Hi, Jamison. I'm Diane, the paramedic in charge of your transport today."

"He can't talk," my mom says from across the room.

"Oh, okay," the paramedic says. "Jamison, can you roll on your side for me? We're going to put a tarp under you."

I try to turn over on my own, but I'm too weak. I try again and the paramedic pushes on my back. It hurts but I slowly roll on my side. Then she slides a tarp underneath me and I return to the supine position. I can feel the smooth, thick, cold plastic under my back. Two EMTs then grab the tarp's handles and lift me out of bed. Just like that I'm in the air, detached from my mattress for the first time in months, my body folded into the tarp like a hot dog in a bun.

I'm carried downstairs and feel someone's hands on the back of my neck as my head bobs over the edge of the tarp. The hands steady my head all the way down the stairs until I'm outside. Then I feel a soft, warm breeze on my skin. I hear birds chirping and, for a second, my feet rub against a bush. I feel the leafy foliage on my toes. I may not be able to see my surroundings, but I can touch and hear them. And damn does it feel good. Being outside for the first time in months is the greatest thing ever. It's bewildering and humbling, exciting and mystifying. I feel like I'm a child again, experiencing things for the first time.

The crew puts me on a gurney and rolls me in the back of the ambulance. The paramedic hooks me up to a saline drip and a machine monitoring my vital signs. I lift the layers from my eyes again to catch a glimpse of my surroundings, but as soon as I do, I'm blinded by sunlight glaring through the windows in the ambulance. It makes my symptoms flare, so I cover my eyes and rely on my hearing instead.

The fifteen-minute drive is mostly silent except for the sound of the blood pressure cuff on my arm filling with air and the ambulance driver talking on the radio. I hear him say, "We've got a twenty-six-year-old male with a possible UTI, and his mom says he has chronic fatigue syndrome." The man's voice takes on a skeptical tone, as if to say, *is chronic fatigue syndrome really a thing?*

The ambulance pulls up to the hospital, and once again I feel fresh air as I'm wheeled inside. Then someone moves me to a bed, and, as far as I can tell, leaves me alone in what is, judging by the loud noises and bright lights, a very crowded emergency room. Someone, probably a nurse, hooks me up to a heart monitor and saline drip. IV saline means more liquids in my already full bladder, a giant water balloon that can't drain. I feel around on the hospital bed for a urinal or some sort of container so I can try to squeeze out some piss, but I find nothing.

This situation is unfamiliar and scary. I'm alone in a busy hospital with a bladder about to burst, and I can't see anything because the lights are too bright.

"Do you need to pee?" I hear my mom say. I didn't even know she was here. But I'm glad she is. She slides a plastic urinal next to me. I grab her hand and give it a little squeeze. "Your dad just got here. He's getting you some food."

I put a few short spurts of pee in the urinal, hardly making room in my bulging bladder. Then my dad arrives with some soup and a straw. I drink the warm butternut squash soup as someone new walks up to my bed.

"Hi, folks. I'm Matt, your nurse," the man says. "And this is . . . Jamison, UTI, chronic fatigue. Okay."

I can't see the nurse, but I assume he's reading from an intake form. When he finishes going over my paperwork, I feel him attach a plastic hospital bracelet to my wrist.

Not another damn hospital bracelet.

"He's having trouble urinating and it's painful," my mom says. "He also has a fever."

"Okay, we're going to do a urine test, then the doctor will let you know the results. Is that good to go?" I peek at the nurse pointing to the urinal I just used.

"Is it enough?" my dad asks, handing the nurse the urinal.

"We'll make it work," he replies.

At least an hour goes by, and finally a doctor stops by to see me. I peek at his face, and he looks like he's only a few years older than me. The doctor goes through a typical patient exam with no concessions to my delicate condition. He takes off my eye mask and sunglasses. The artificial lighting in the room burns my brain as he tells me, with a mocking tone, how beautiful my eyes are and how I shouldn't keep them hidden. I want to punch him. Then he shines a bright flashlight on my pupils, and I want to punch him even more. I cover my eyes back up, and the doctor checks my mouth and gives equally mocking praise to my teeth. Meanwhile the residual effects from the harsh lights bring on tremors. My body trembles as the doctor finishes the checkup, and he says he'll be back when the lab results are ready.

Another hour goes by before my dad flags down the nurse.

"Any word yet?" he asks. "My son's in a lot of pain. He can't urinate."

"Uh, yeah. His lab results aren't terrible," the nurse says.

"What do you mean they aren't terrible?" my dad asks.

"I'll let the doctor talk to you about it."

Half an hour later, the doctor finally returns with the results.

"Okay . . . I can't make a definitive diagnosis because not enough bacteria showed up in Jamison's urine," the doctor says. "But I suspect it's a UTI. So I'm going to write him a prescription for three days of an antibiotic. Your GP can fill the rest. For now just drink lots of fluids to flush the bacteria out."

Are you kidding me? This guy's a fucking quack. Out of every-thing at his disposal, he does a simple urine test and tells you to drink water when your bladder is clogged and about to fucking explode. Did he actually graduate from medical school, or was he too busy commenting on everyone's eyes?

"Excuse me but he can't see a general practitioner," my mom says.

"Of course he can," the doctor says. "In his condition, he especially needs to see a GP for regular checkups, and so he can start physical therapy."

"He's too sick to travel," my mom says. "How's he going to get to a doctor's office in his condition?"

"He traveled here, didn't he?" the doctor asks rhetorically.

"This is an emergency," my mom replies. "It took five people just to get him in the ambulance."

"That's precisely why he should be working on rehab with a physical therapist," the doctor argues. "He needs to get his strength back, so he doesn't need people to carry him."

"He's too sick to rehab."

"I doubt that," the doctor says.

"Look at him—he can't even sit up," my mom says. Her voice gets louder and starts to quaver.

"As I said, he needs to work with a physical therapist."

"This is pointless," my mom shouts. But the hospital is so loud and buzzing with activity that her raised voice is barely noticeable. "I'm not going to stand here and talk to you about physical therapy when my son is so sick he can't speak or chew food. Please call an ambulance so we can leave."

"His insurance won't cover that," the doctor replies.

"What do you mean his insurance won't cover it? Who are you to tell me what his insurance won't cover?" my mom says.

"Chronic fatigue is not a legitimate condition. It's not like someone who was in a car accident or someone with a bad heart. Those people require an ambulance. He does not."

"You really want to have this conversation with me?" my mom says.

"I'm just doing my job," the doctor insists.

"No, you're not just doing your job," my mom fires back. "If you were, my son would be able to urinate, and his fever would be gone. Your job is to treat him, but you won't do that because you're too ignorant." My mom pauses and I hear her take a long breath. "Unless you want him to stay here, I suggest you get us an ambulance now."

I thought my mom had reached her breaking point already, but I was wrong. She's not broken. She's just warming up. She's finally found a recipient worthy of the intense anger that's been building up inside her these last few months. I'm grateful that she's sticking up for me. If she weren't, I would just have to lie here on this stupid hospital bed while this idiot doctor treats me like a hypochondriac.

The doctor finally calls an ambulance, and he and my mom acrimoniously end the argument. Before I leave, a nurse walks over and asks me to sign a form. I grab her pen and feel around on the paper with my eyes still covered. Holding the pen is painful and weakens my grip, so I grasp it with both hands and blindly scribble a couple squiggly lines.

The ambulance arrives, and a paramedic puts me on a gurney and takes me home, where I'm put back on my tiny twin mattress. For some stupid reason, the first thing I do once I'm back in bed is drink water, just as the ER doctor ordered. Within minutes my bladder expands even more. Now it looks like I have a pasta strainer sticking out of my belly.

I'm in excruciating pain and the tremors are more intense than ever, shooting through my entire body. I start to make the same whimpering sound I made a few months ago after I spilled piss all over my bed. Now I would gladly dump a whole quart of piss on my bed, if only I could get it out of my bladder.

My mom hears the whimpering and comes to check on me. She takes my temperature—102.1 degrees. She gives me Tylenol and sits next to my bed, waiting for my fever to break. But it doesn't break. It keeps surging higher.

I grab a urinal and push down on my bladder until a long spurt of pee is forced out. I do it again but get tired. My mom takes over and starts pushing down on my bladder. We keep switching off until a pint or so is in the urinal beside me. Finally my body relaxes, and my fever goes down. My mom looks relieved as she puts her hand on my wrist, where my new hospital bracelet is attached.

"Do you want me to take that off?" she asks. I give her a thumbs up. "I can put it with the other one you saved from your car accident . . ."

I shake my head and give her a thumbs down. I don't need another reminder of a bad day. My mom snaps the bracelet off my wrist and throws it in the trash, then she leaves me to rest.

As I lie in bed, the darkness of my room surrounding me, I start to think about my other hospital bracelet and what it symbolizes. It's been a long time since I've thought about the car accident. I've done a lot to cope with the trauma, but as my health has declined, it has gotten more difficult to stay in touch with that part of my life. That's one of the most frustrating things about being sick: the illness consumes everything in its path and leaves little time or energy to think about anything other than survival. With the illness raging inside my body, it has been nearly impossible for me to focus on the car accident. But when my mom mentioned my hospital bracelet, thoughts flooded my mind.

The car accident was a big, ugly, traumatic part of my life. And for a time, a year and a half or so, I thought it was going to be the most traumatic part of my life. But I knew I could handle it. I knew I could cope with it and move on. And I did. I talked about the trauma with friends, family, and a support group. I took out my frustrations in the gym and eventually found Ellen, the therapist who taught me the most about my trauma. But as much as she showed me, neither she, nor I, knew what lay ahead. The trauma we were talking about then wasn't as intense and definitely not as chronic as the trauma I now face with my illness.

Sure, one day six years ago, I was stuck on a bridge next to a burning body and it was fucking terrible, probably the worst thing I could have imagined at the time. But it wasn't the same as what I've experienced with my illness. The accident was a singular traumatic event, a wound that has been healing and will continue to heal as time goes on. But now I have to live with a new type of trauma, a more continuous kind. Having a severe chronic illness is the kind of trauma that never heals; it's a wound that just keeps reopening and getting bigger. The trauma of lying in my own shit every time I have a bowel movement and spilling bottles of piss all over my bed while not being able to call for help is more traumatic than ten of my car accidents. And I say that not to minimize being in a car accident but to illustrate that it's a different kind of trauma, a more acute kind.

As much as I'd like to say that I've fully recovered from the car accident, I'm not going to because I don't know if I have. I do know that I've reached a point where I rarely think about the accident but for an occasional reminder, like my mom asking about the hospital bracelet. I don't have flashbacks or imagine car crashes anymore, which seems like progress, but I honestly don't know if it's because I've dealt with those issues properly, or if they've merely disappeared now that I'm too sick to drive. Similarly, I don't know if I've forgotten about the man who died in the accident because I've come to terms with ending his life or because I never knew him, never saw a face to go with the life that was lost. And as much as I'd like to dig deeper into why he was stopped in the middle of the highway at the top of a steep bridge, I'm too busy trying to get my health back, too consumed with trying to heal the reoccurring trauma of my illness.

I may never figure these things out. In fact, I probably won't. But that's okay. I may be sick and have experienced enough trauma for a hundred lifetimes, but I'm still here, fighting for each day.

After a few hours of lying in the darkness, thinking about the car accident, it once again fades to the recesses of my mind, and the illness takes over. My mom checks on me and realizes that my bladder is full again and the fever is back. She panics and calls a friend at her work who knows a doctor at the local health clinic. He agrees to come to the house and examine me.

After checking my vital signs, he turns me over and gives me a prostate exam, which is, to put it mildly, not the best experience. But it is necessary because the doctor concludes that I have a swollen prostate gland, not a urinary tract infection. Now I'm sort of glad the ER doctor didn't do his job. I would have hated that smug shithead sticking his fingers up my ass. This doctor is more respectful and actually knows what he's doing. He says the swollen prostate was probably caused by lying in the supine position too long. It seems the antidepressant I took made me so immobile that my prostate got stuck in a bad position, which is why it's inflamed and has blocked off the flow of my urine.

Before leaving, the doctor prescribes Flomax, a medication to reduce the swelling. He tells me to take it until I get some strength back and can move around enough to take pressure off my prostate. A few hours after taking the medication, the problem is solved. My fever is gone, and finally I can pee freely again.

CHAPTER 47

The Physical Therapist

July 7, 2015

Claire has come to visit, and despite being pregnant, she's handling most of my care until my mom can hire a permanent caregiver. Since her arrival, Claire has introduced me to several things that make it easier for me to communicate and improve my quality of life. She bought me a buzzer when I spill a urinal and need to call someone to help me clean it up. Because I'm still too sick to use my phone, when I've needed help I've had to torturously wait for someone to check on me; either that, or when I've been really desperate, I'd push a heavy object off my bed so it would *thump* on the floor. Now I just press a call button, and it rings throughout the house.

When someone answers the buzzer, Claire has taught me an alphabet spelling system to communicate. A few years ago, she learned it while taking care of a man with ALS. I visited her when she was caring for him. At the time, the spelling system seemed confusing, but it was his only way to communicate.

Now I find myself in a similar situation—the spelling system is my only reliable way of communicating.

When I first saw Claire use the spelling system, she started by holding up a small whiteboard with the alphabet written on it in rows, each row starting with a vowel. Then she called out the vowels—*A, E, I,* and when she got to *O,* the man with ALS blinked, the only voluntary movement he could make. Then Claire named the vowel and consonants in that row—*O, P, Q,* and when she got to *R,* the man blinked again, signaling that *R* was the first letter of the word he wanted to spell. As complicated as it is, at least the spelling system isn't entirely unfamiliar to me, which has made it easier to master.

Claire has also made shaving easier for me by using an electric razor. It's fairly quiet, a noise level I can handle, but the weight is heavy, so Claire has to hold it for me while I guide her hand around my face. It's awkward but still easier than trying to use a sharp manual razor.

Another issue that I've been dealing with is my disappearing body weight. I'm gaunt and malnourished, even more so than when I first got sick. My ribs poke out of my torso. There's little fat or muscle anywhere on my body. I'm just skin and bones.

Most of the weight that I've lost is from inactivity and being restricted to a liquid diet of mainly protein shakes. I've probably lost more than thirty pounds since January, which would put my body weight around one hundred and ten pounds, though it's impossible to say for sure because I'm too weak to stand on a scale. Regardless of how much weight I've lost, just by looking at my body, it's clear that I'm not getting enough nutrients.

Thankfully Claire and my mom are helping me put on weight. They have created a palatable menu of liquid meals consisting of dishes like scrambled eggs and lobster ravioli, which they purée in a blender with broth. My dad has also contributed to the menu with a Greek yogurt and nut butter shake that is filling and tastes good.

The protein in these meals is crucial for me to put on weight and to regain my strength. But it's also a reminder that, for such a long time, I've been obsessed with building muscle, and now I must accept the fact that the muscular physique I spent countless hours building in the gym is gone. And not just a little gone. It's nonexistent.

Five years ago, I was a tan bodybuilder who could lift over four hundred pounds. Two years ago, I was still tan, if a bit flabby, and could barely lift forty pounds. Now, the sickest I've ever been, I have the complexion of a fifteenth-century European monarch, and I can't even lift a glass of water. My muscles struggle with the lightest weight. I wish I could strengthen them, but I don't have the energy or ability to do any exercises. And it's not as if my inactivity has made me this weak. As Dr. Peterson said, this isn't deconditioning, this illness impairs my energy and strength production.

Nevertheless, I need to maintain what little strength I have left, so I'm following the ER doctor's orders to work with a physical therapist. I don't expect the physical therapy to do much. I know it won't treat my illness. But maybe if I pace myself, it'll help with my strength. And even if it doesn't, I have to do it to qualify for disability benefits, which I need to pay my bills.

Today is my first session with the physical therapist. When she arrives, Claire is battling morning sickness but manages to welcome the woman inside. They talk for a bit, but all I can hear are murmurs. Then, surprisingly, Claire raises her voice and shouts, "I don't like being talked to like an idiot," which is followed by the slamming of a door in the back of the house.

Well, at least things are starting off well.

I hear Claire stomping around outside. Then, a few minutes later, my mom comes home and welcomes the physical therapist into my dark cave of a room. The athletic-looking woman, wearing workout clothes and a stopwatch, quickly gets to work instructing me to lift my arms above my head. I give her a thumbs down. Then, without acknowledging my hand gesture, she asks if she can lift my arm for me. I agree, thinking she'll be gentle. She's not gentle.

In one swift motion, she lifts my right arm above my head. A sharp, burning pain shoots through my right shoulder. I start to whimper and tremble, but the physical therapist is completely oblivious to my condition. She grabs my left arm and repeats the motion. Now the pain jolts through my left shoulder. I'm able to get my arm free from the physical therapist's grasp, but she continues, grabbing my right arm again. My mom sees the pain on my face and cuts her off. She resists and asks me if I'd like to continue. I shake my head and she looks surprised, if not insulted. The physical therapist continues to hold a firm grip on my arm, and my mom once again steps in and, this time, physically removes the woman's hand from my arm.

Finally my mom ushers the physical therapist toward the bedroom door. Before walking out, the woman says, "See you tomorrow, Jamison."

You can't see her tomorrow. You can't move your arms. It's going to take you weeks to recover from this lady's hyper-aggressive bullshit.

Several minutes later, Claire walks in with an angry look on her face.

"She was a real piece of work," Claire says. I nod my head and make a plank with my hand, the signal I use to initiate the new spelling system.

"You want to use the spelling board?" Claire asks.

I give a thumbs up. She shows me a whiteboard with the alphabet written on it, like the one she used for the man with ALS.

"Okay, *A* . . . *E* . . . *I*—"

I give her another thumbs up.

"Is it . . . *I* . . . *J* . . . *K* . . . *L* . . . *M* . . . *N*—"

I give a thumbs up.

"*N* is the first letter?" Claire asks. I nod. "Second letter . . ." She holds up the whiteboard again. "*A* . . . *E* . . . *I* . . . *O*—"

I give another thumbs up.

"*O*—" Claire starts to say, then I give a thumbs up. "Is the word *no*?" I nod. "Is there another word?" I nod again. "Okay, first word is *no*. Now the second word: *A* . . . *E* . . . *I*—"

I give a thumbs up.

"*I* . . . *J* . . . *K* . . . *L* . . . *M*—"

I give her another thumbs up. My hands are throbbing with pain from moving my thumbs. I try to expedite the process by making an *O* shape with my hand.

"*O*? So, the first letter of the second word is *M* and the second letter is *O*?"

I give a thumbs up.

"All right. Third letter: *A* . . . *E* . . . *I* . . . *O*—"

I give Claire another thumbs up as my hands continue to burn with inflammation.

"*O* . . . *P* . . . *Q* . . . *R*—"

I give a thumbs up.

"*M* . . . *O* . . . *R*? Is the second word *More*?" Claire asks, filling in the last letter. I nod. "What was the first word again? *No*? *No more*?"

I give a triumphant thumbs up.

"You mean no more physical therapy?" she asks. I make a praying gesture with my hands. "Oh, don't worry, brother. That crazy lady won't be coming back."

I sigh in relief, then a sudden wave of sadness hits me. I'm not exactly sure what triggers the feeling, probably the combative physical therapist who yanked on my arms, or it could have been what she symbolizes—the person I used to be. As a fitness instructor, I had a job similar to hers. Seeing her workout clothes and stopwatch made me miss my old job and how capable I used to be. Back then I would have loved to do some physical therapy. Okay, maybe I wouldn't have loved it, because who loves physical therapy? But at least I would have been good at it. I would have kicked some physical therapy ass.

Now the reality is that I can't even do basic arm movements without getting injured and making myself sicker. And I'm sick enough as it is, so sick that my family has to apply for disability benefits for me.

Being labeled as disabled stirs a feeling of grief inside me—I'm mourning the loss of my fit, healthy self all over again. It's been years since I've had a healthy body, and now, in such a debilitated state, I feel a profound sense of hopelessness.

It must show on my face because Claire looks at me and asks, "What's wrong, brother?"

I take a deep breath and point to my head, then give a thumbs down, meaning, "I'm having bad thoughts." I'm tired of fighting, tired of punching an invisible opponent, shadow boxing an illness that I barely know anything about, an illness that nobody seems to take seriously. Somehow this ridiculous disease has managed to take me down and, at the same time, evade every doctor I've seen. I'm done with it all. I don't want to fight this battle anymore.

"Your thoughts are bad?" Claire asks, recognizing my hand gestures.

I give a thumbs up, then spell out *suicide*.

"You want to kill yourself?" Claire asks. "Then what're you gonna do? You'll be gone." She pauses. "Listen, I know this fucking sucks, brother, but you are doing better, and you will get better. It's a bad situation, but just remember this is only one bad day. It'll pass. "

Claire's words are comforting and make me realize that, as hopeless as I feel, I just don't have the courage to end my life. No matter how miserable things get, I would be too scared to kill myself, too afraid that I'd botch an attempt. And then there's my fear that, if I were successful, there wouldn't be an afterlife, and I'd prematurely fade into oblivion. But most of all, I can't kill myself because there's still a chance that my health and quality of life will improve. As long as I'm alive, there will always be that possibility, and I must cling to it. I must keep going, keep fighting this evil illness and hold out hope that my health will someday improve.

CHAPTER 48

A Tragic Manscaping Accident

August 28, 2015

At least a dozen people have taken care of me while I've been stuck here in bed. Most have been family, like Claire, who has now returned home. In the brief time since Claire left, other caregivers have been hired, then fired. One caregiver kept calling in sick, forcing my mom to miss work to take care of me. Another caregiver treated the job like a volunteer position, essentially making her own rules and schedule.

One of the biggest issues my mom has had with hiring caregivers is the cost. She's been hiring them through an agency that charges twenty-five dollars an hour, more than my mom makes as a teacher, and less than half of which goes to the actual caregiver. The worst part is that the agency calls itself a charity.

Luckily, we've moved on from the "charity" and have hired a caregiver directly. Her name is Randi. She's the same age as my mom, and although her heart seems to be in the right place, she often lacks tact. This became clear one day when I pointed to my throat because I was choking on a pill and needed her help. After several wrong guesses, Randi gave up and asked if she should get a knife and slit my throat.

Although my irritation with her is partially the result of needing to unload my anger, she is, at the very least, an odd person. Randi can be bossy and abrasive, and she assumes her way is always best. She doesn't ask what I like to eat; she just makes what she wants. Then she talks my head into a dizzying state, giving me discourses on the weather outside compared to the temperature inside, and how having my window open disrupts the balance.

Caregiving is one of the hardest professions there is. It's a messy, underpaid job, and to be honest, it's one I could never do. Caregivers deserve every cent that I can't afford to pay them. Because I don't have an income, my mom has had to pay my caregivers, including Randi who makes fifteen dollars an hour, plus a daily stipend for her commute.

Today Randi will be training a new caregiver, who I secretly hope will replace her. My mom left for work a while ago, and now I'm home alone, waiting for Randi and her trainee to show up. I feel a bowel movement coming on, the timing of which could not be worse. I'm alone with no one to help me. There's a hand towel on my bed, which I grab and shuffle under my hip. Then I turn on my side, handle my business, and wait for Randi to arrive.

After several minutes of lying next to a pile of shit, I hear the front door open and press my buzzer. Randi and the new caregiver enter my dark room, and I show them two fingers.

"Jamison, my eyes are still adjusting to the dark. Is that two fingers?" Randi forcefully grabs my fingers, squelching what little strength I have in my hand. I click the roof of my mouth as confirmation. "When he shows you two fingers, that's the sign for a bowel movement," Randi explains to her trainee, as I continue to lie in my own feces.

Randi grabs an absorbent pad and I think about trying to tell her that I've already finished the bowel movement but decide to save my energy because she'll eventually notice the mess I've made. She must. But she doesn't. Randi blindly shoves the pad under my hip, taking a log of my shit with it. She continues by sliding a garbage bag, and yes, more shit under my legs. It's beyond humiliating. It is probably the grossest thing to ever happen to me, but for some inexplicable reason I stay calm and let the two caregivers leave the room. A few seconds later I press the buzzer, then they return and Randi grabs the empty garbage bag.

"Are you done?" she asks, feeling around the bag. "There's nothing here."

I lean forward and point under my hips. She feels around under me. "Oh, wait, oh no. I see what happened."

Randi helps me turn over and begins to slowly clean me up, frequently pausing to instruct her trainee. At one point she casually tells the new caregiver, "He likes his anus really clean."

Does that mean she doesn't like her anus clean? No wonder she lacks tact, she's walking around with an itchy asshole.

If Randi smearing shit on me and talking about my anus wasn't bad enough, now I need her help with another delicate personal problem. I've had a nasty rash around my scrotum for weeks, probably from the lack of ventilation that comes with being stuck on a mattress all the time.

I've asked Randi to trim the hair around the rash so I can put ointment on it. For some reason, the danger of using scissors on the most sensitive part of my body in a dark room doesn't register with me, or Randi. So we proceed. The first few snips are clean, but suddenly I feel a sharp blade, two of them actually, slicing the skin on my scrotum. Blood drips down my thighs. I can't see it, but I can feel the warm, viscous liquid oozing out of me. And now the combination of darkness, a sharp object, and my scrotum seems like the dumbest idea in the world.

Randi frantically apologizes while I continue to bleed. As news headlines of a bedridden man bleeding to death in a tragic manscaping accident flash in my head, Randi gives me a cloth to stop the bleeding. She seems distraught, as much as someone can in the dark, and my scrotum, well, it feels like a swollen, lopsided pouch of fiery flesh. This is not the first time Randi has damaged my private parts. Last week, she mistook my genitals for a washcloth, pinching and yanking on them, as she tried to toss the washcloth in the laundry hamper.

I do my best to continue tending to my hygiene, but the pain and embarrassment, the shame and indignity of failing to do simple tasks even with the help of other people, makes me want to scream. So, when Randi asks if I want help cleaning my "shaft," that's exactly what I do. I turn away from her and pretend to go to sleep. I've had enough of her talking about my *anus*, *scrotum*, and *shaft* for one day.

CHAPTER 49

Friends

September 12, 2015

One of the hardest parts of being bedridden is losing contact with friends. It's been about a year since I've seen any of mine. That is, until recently. Now that I've recovered from the prostatitis and can move around my bed with small amounts of strength, some of my friends have come to visit. Many of them have said how peaceful and calming my dark room is, but it's only peaceful and calming to them. To me, it's a lonely, isolated prison cell that I desperately want to escape.

My friends serve as a somber reminder of the difference between me and a healthy person. Some of them ask me, "How are you feeling today?" I know the question comes from a good place, but the last thing I want to talk about is how I feel, especially when I have to use the spelling system to do it.

Thomas, my old roommate from Sonoma State, is one of my friends who recently visited. The moment he entered my dark room, I was reminded of how present and supportive he's been during some of the most challenging moments of my life. He was there the day I first got sick after working out. He was there a year later when I had to leave Sonoma and say goodbye to the life I had created for myself. And finally, he was there for me just a few days ago as I lay in bed unable to sit up or take part in our usual banter. Though, there was one moment during the visit that felt just like old times.

When Thomas walked in my room, I felt like making him laugh, so I took the sheet off my legs, revealing my pasty thighs. Then I used the spelling system to say, "I'm naked." We both laughed, or rather Thomas laughed, and I tried to but ended up wincing because laughing feels like someone jumping up and down on my chest.

I enjoyed Thomas's visit, but when he told me that he has now started working as a fitness instructor, I felt defeated. There he was—healthy, strong, and essentially living my old life, the life I've lost and miss so much. Knowing that he's doing the things I love made my life as a fitness instructor feel so distant and my current life as a sick and disabled person feel so unbearable.

As envious as I was of his success, seeing Thomas reminded me of how close we've been over the last several years. It made me think of the last night we spent in Sonoma before we moved out of our house. All our belongings had been packed away in boxes or piled against the walls. We had no TV or video games to occupy our time, so we spent the whole night talking about what we wanted to do with the rest of our lives. He told me that he wanted to work in the fitness industry, and I told him that I wanted to get my health back so we could open a gym together. We talked for such a long time that I eventually fell asleep. I expected that Thomas would go back to his room, but when I woke up a few hours later, he was still there, sleeping at the foot of my bed. There was something about that moment, seeing Thomas sleeping near me on our last night as roommates, that made me cherish his friendship more than ever. Now here we are, under sadder circumstances but just as closely bonded.

Before Thomas left, he talked about *Forgotten Plague*, the ME/CFS documentary that I'm featured in. I haven't been able to watch it, but Thomas said that my current condition—bedridden and unable to speak or eat solid food—bears striking similarities to another patient in the film—Whitney Dafoe, the gaunt man that Ryan Prior, one of the film's directors, told me about a few years ago.

Occasionally my mom updates me on Whitney's condition, which she reads about online. His entire family, like mine, has been consumed by this illness. His mother, Janet, is his main caregiver; his sister, Ashley, helps with fundraising and community organizing for ME/CFS; and his father, Ron, a geneticist at Stanford University, is researching severely ill patients with the help of a Bay Area organization called Open Medicine. The medical director of the Open Medicine Clinic, Dr. David Kaufman, treats many ME/CFS patients. I'm currently on the waiting list for a phone appointment with him. I don't have much faith in doctors anymore, but because he works with severely ill patients, I have hope that he can help me regain some of the health I've lost.

CHAPTER 50

You Want a Kiss?

October 12, 2015

Another one of my friends is coming to visit. Sasha is going to be here for a few weeks, mainly to help my mom with moving into a new house. My mom bought the house back in April, but I've been too sick to do the move. Now that my condition has stabilized a bit and I can handle a short ambulance ride, we are moving forward with our plans to live in a house better suited for both of us.

Sasha arrives and walks into my room after talking with my mom downstairs. It's the first time I've seen her since she visited me in Santa Cruz.

"I missed you," she says with a nervous quaver in her voice.

I give her a big smile and point to my mouth, my way of asking her to talk to me.

"You want a kiss?" she asks, sounding unsure of her question and even more unsure of my potential answer. I almost give her a thumbs up, but instead I awkwardly point to my mouth again and wait for her to make another guess.

"I don't know what that means," Sasha says. "Let me go ask your mom."

Sasha walks downstairs and returns after a brief conversation with my mom.

"Okay, you want me to talk to you? Not kiss you?"

I shrug my shoulders and give her a flirtatious smile.

"Are you sure you want me to talk when we could just make out?" she says.

I shrug again and smile.

We continue to flirt for a while, then she goes to bed, and for a long time, I stay awake thinking about the possibility of finally, after all this time, kissing Sasha.

CHAPTER 51

Boyfriend

November 5, 2015

Today I have a phone appointment with Dr. David Kaufman from the Open Medicine Clinic. I'm not feeling well enough to participate in the phone call, so this appointment is going to be unlike any I've had before.

It starts with the doctor calling my mom, who's recording the conversation for me to listen to when I'm feeling better. The two of them talk about my recent blood work, which was done a week ago by a wonderful nurse who was able to draw more than fifteen vials of blood without throwing a single punch to my arm.

It's bizarre to not be involved in my own doctor's appointment, but because I'm too weak to travel to see Dr. Kaufman, it's the only way I can get the treatment I need. For the duration of the call, I remain in my room, intermittently listening to my mom talking on the phone just outside my door.

The call ends and my mom gives me a summary of the conversation. She says the doctor is going to give me some new treatments to try, and I can listen to the recording of the call when I'm up for it. For now, though, I rest.

That is, until Sasha walks in the room with the usual bounce in her step, wearing workout attire under a jacket she borrowed from my closet. It's from my high school days and has my name embroidered on the back.

I'm glad Sasha is here. In the weeks that she's been visiting, she has kept me company, and my mom has really put her to work, packing my stuff and even shoveling gravel for our driveway.

"Hi, you," Sasha says, sitting next to my bed. "How's it going?"

I give a thumbs up, then point at her.

"Me?" Sasha asks. I nod. "Oh. I'm good. You would have been proud of me today—I got a gym membership. Now I can work out while I'm here. I did the treadmill this morning. Boy, it wore me out."

I smile, then scoot over and pat the bed.

"You want me to lay with you?" Sasha asks.

I give a thumbs up.

"Okay, uh, but let me go shower first."

Sasha returns, smelling fresh and wearing pajamas.

"Okay, I'm ready," she says, lying down beside me. For the first time in at least a year, I have an attractive, young woman in my bed, and I couldn't be happier about it. Sharing a pillow with Sasha makes me feel alive. I wish it were under healthier circumstances, and with fewer articles of clothing between us, but seeing as I'm too sick to do anything sexual, I'll settle for some cuddling. Besides, Sasha's elbow is resting on the pillow in front of her face, blocking any attempts I could make at trying to kiss her. Instead I just softly hold her hand. But when I do, she looks at me with a worried expression on her face.

"I need to tell you something," Sasha says. "I should have told you already. I don't know why I didn't, but, um." She pauses. "I have a boyfriend."

It feels like I was just punched in the chest. For once I'm glad I can't speak. If I could, I'd probably overreact and say something stupid that I would regret. I'm not entirely sure why it's so devastating for me to find out that Sasha has a boyfriend. It has, after all, been two years since we've seen each other. It was naïve of me to think that she would still be single, and quixotic of me to think that she would come visit and fall in love with a sick guy who can't walk or talk.

CHAPTER 52

Free

November 15, 2015

Sasha walks into my room and sits next to me with an anxious look on her face.

"Okay, sweet boy, you need to make a decision," Sasha says.

I point to my temple.

"Thinking? You're still thinking about it?" she asks.

I shake my head and point to Sasha.

"Me? What am I thinking?" she asks. I make a hand gesture that means her guess was almost right. "Oh, what do I think you should do?"

I nod and smirk.

"Um, well, I think we should get you out of here. It's dark outside, so you won't need to cover your eyes. Maybe they'll even leave us alone in the back of the ambulance to have some fun."

I decide to go for it and give a thumbs up. Sasha relays the message to my mom, who makes a non-emergency call for an ambulance. Soon there's another band of first responders beside my bed, trying once again to maneuver a tarp under my frail body and carry me onto a gurney.

This time it's Sasha who holds my head bobbing over the tarp while I'm carried outside. There, for only the second time in a year, I feel fresh open air. It's just as invigorating as the last time but short lived.

I'm put on the gurney and into the back of the ambulance. Sasha holds my hand while she awkwardly crouches next to me. From the driver's seat, I hear the voice of the same driver from the ambulance ride I took back in June. Then I feel the paramedic's hands wrap a blood pressure cuff around my arm.

The ambulance takes us up several steep mountain roads, and we get lost a few times, but eventually we arrive at the new house perched atop a mountain ridge overlooking the Central Valley. I have no idea what the new house or its view look like, but apparently they're both pretty great. When the paramedic wheels me onto the deck, I hear him say, "Wow, look at that view."

The only view I can see is a ceiling as I'm shoveled onto my new bed. This changes when everyone leaves and Sasha crawls into bed with me.

"Now that wasn't too bad," she says.

I look at her cockeyed.

"Okay, okay, we did get lost, but you're fine."

I look at her even more cockeyed.

"Ah, okay, you're not fine, but you're alive."

I smile politely.

"So how come you haven't kissed me yet?" Sasha asks, shocking me as only she can.

The word *boyfriend* comes to mind, but I take the question as rhetorical and a direct challenge, maybe even an invitation. The idea of kissing Sasha consumes my thoughts. Time seems to stop as I move to Sasha's side of the pillow. My hand touches her cheek, making my brain buzz and my heart thump loudly throughout my body.

My lungs start to burn, and my breathing becomes labored, reminding me of all the times late at night when I would pop in my earbuds and sprint up and down the steps on the Sonoma State campus. My heart is still thumping loudly and I feel little tremors starting to rip through my body. I consider retreating, but then something sort of magical happens: my pulse slows and the tremors stop.

I gently press my hand against Sasha's cheek, tucking my fingers behind her ear. Then I softly press my lips to hers. They fit together perfectly. There's no awkward fumbling around, no bonked heads or poked eyes, just a well-placed kiss, and oh what a kiss. There's no champagne or fireworks, but realization of a long overdue connection between us. Kissing Sasha feels freeing to me. No longer am I a prisoner in my own body, stuck in a bed within a dark room of an unfamiliar house. I'm free—a genie released from his lamp, a bird with a healed wing. For a fleeting moment, I'm free of the muscle pain and debilitating weakness, free of the horrible nausea and scary tremors rattling my body. Never did I think kissing would have such a tantalizing effect at this point in my life. But it does and I don't question it.

I know Sasha is destined to be my friend, not my girlfriend. I know she will soon return to her job and her boyfriend, but that's okay. She has given me such a gift. I'm thankful for the moments we've had together. When we first met at the coffee shop near Sonoma State, she made me feel normal in a way only a caring, healthy person can make a lonely, sick person feel. When she came to visit me in Santa Cruz, she helped me, however unknowingly, examine the lack of companionship in my life. Now, she has given me the genuine affection and intimacy that I've craved for such a long time, when no one else would and when I needed it most. She has allowed my needs, the needs of her severely ill friend, to supersede the obligations of her life. She has put her career and relationship, and probably countless other things, on hold to make me feel loved. For that, I will always be grateful.

But, as it seems, neither of us is ready to return to reality just yet. After our first kiss, Sasha and I breathe each other in as our lips part, and we return to our respective ends of the pillow, our eyes nervously fixed on one another like teenagers on a first date. I take a deep breath and calm my body. I think about how wonderful this moment is, and how it seems to transcend everything that's plaguing my body. I collect myself for a few more seconds, then motion for Sasha to come back to me because I just want to feel free a little longer.

YEAR 6

Answers

CHAPTER 53

A Bit Better

February 18, 2016

I'm about to relisten to the recording of the phone call my mom had with Dr. Kaufman, in case I missed something the first time I listened to it back in November. At first, I didn't have much faith that the doctor could help. After all, none of the other doctors that I've seen have made any sustainable improvement in my health. But because I've been so sick and in such desperate need of medical care, I've put myself at the mercy of Dr. Kaufman's treatments, which he has prescribed based on my lab work, despite having never seen me in person.

To my surprise and delight, the treatments seem to be working. I'm feeling a bit better. The improvements have been subtle: I'm not as sensitive to light, and my pain and weakness have gradually decreased. As terrifying as it was to have my body fail, seeing it start working again has been inspiring.

Right now the doctor has me taking four huge antiviral pills to fight the active viruses he discovered in my blood work.

He also has me on a steroid called hydrocortisone for my low cortisol levels, and a slew of vitamins to supplement my liquid diet until I start eating solid food again. Soon he's planning to prescribe me subcutaneous vitamin injections and daily infusions through a foot-long IV catheter inserted into a large vein that runs from my biceps to my heart.

It's a lot to wrap my head around, but perhaps there's even more. I start the recording:

Dr. Kaufman: Hi Kathleen. Are you alone, or is Jamison able to hear me?

Kathleen: He's not able to hear. I can ask if he's up for it, but I don't know that he would be.

Dr. Kaufman: Okay. This is our first follow-up since Jamison's initial lab work, even though I have not actually seen him, or you, for that matter. So let me just read you what I wrote for him. I want to make sure I got his history right. Okay?

Kathleen: Okay.

Dr. Kaufman: Jamison is a twenty-seven-year-old bedridden male. In June of 2009, he was in a fatal motor vehicle accident but was not seriously injured. In November of 2010, he had mono. About two weeks later, he developed tachycardia, a rapid heart rate, near fainting, malaise, chills, nausea, brain fog, disorientation, muscle aches, and pains while working out. He was employed as a personal trainer and ran a boot camp at the time.

His symptoms increased progressively and grew to include photophobia, sound sensitivity, and vertigo. In 2011, he was diagnosed with chronic fatigue syndrome, and then in 2012, he was seen by Dan Peterson.

There was some further improvement, but ultimately he remained chronically ill and could only work on a reduced schedule. In January of 2015, he became progressively worse with flu, fatigue, fever, and he could not move or talk.

Currently, he's one hundred percent bedridden. He cannot stand because of orthostatic intolerance. If the bed is elevated forty-five degrees, he has nausea and gets dizzy in ten seconds. Is that about right?

Kathleen: Yes.

Dr. Kaufman: Okay. I have a note that he's been exposed to dogs and ticks. Did you ever have any cats?

Kathleen: He may have house sat for somebody in Santa Cruz with a cat, but he has never had a cat.

Me (thinking): *Amy strikes again! That damn cat. You probably caught something from all her shit you had to clean up.*

Dr. Kaufman: Okay, fine. Any fleas do you know? Ever been bitten by fleas?

Kathleen: Probably. Family members have some pets.

Dr. Kaufman: All right. Let's go over to his labs. By the way, did the scrotal rash get better?

Kathleen: Yes.

Me (thinking): *That's fucking embarrassing.*

Dr. Kaufman: Great. I assume he's exactly the same . . . bed-bound, miserable?

Kathleen: Yes.

Dr. Kaufman: Okay. We're just going to go through the labs. The first set is totally fine. It's just electrolytes and kidney function, so I think the important thing here is that even though he's not eating well and drinking well, you're doing a great job because he has very good albumin, whIch is a marker for nutrition.

Kathleen : Excellent. Good.

Dr. Kaufman: Next is perhaps one of the most important things: CMV, which stands for Cytomegalovirus. It's a virus that we are all exposed to as children. The antibodies remain positive throughout our life, supposedly, and the virus never disappears from our bodies, so it's latent or locked up in jail so to speak. It can reactivate if there's any immune problems.

Normally the results we see from the antibody tests are either the IgG and the IgM are negative, or more commonly, the IgG is positive, showing prior exposure when we're kids, and the IgM is negative. If you look at Jamison, his IgG is negative, but his IgM is clearly positive. That would suggest that he has ongoing viral activity from this virus. That may be the main cause of what's going on in him. We'll come back to that, but that's a very important result. Next is Epstein-Barr virus, the virus that causes mono. Okay?

Kathleen: Okay.

Dr. Kaufman: There are three different IgG antibody tests that we do for Epstein-Barr. The first one you see is VCA, viral capsid antigen, and that is greater than five. That means it's above the testing limit. The system does not measure above five when it's that high. It's extremely high. It would be reasonable to have it that high if he'd recently had mono, or if he had mono in the last few months, or even maybe in the last year. But if he hasn't had mono in years, this suggests reactivation. Similarly, if you look at the EBNA, Epstein-Barr nuclear antigen, it's the same finding. And the EA, early antigen . . .

Kathleen: Yes . . .

Dr. Kaufman: That's negative. It's usually positive if the reactivation was in the last six to twelve months. This probably means reactivation of the mono virus happened sometime in the last year, maybe a little bit more than a year.

Me (thinking): *That sounds right. It would have been around the time you had to stop working.*

Dr. Kaufman: Now, if you look at the M. pneumoniae test, that's the mycoplasma pneumoniae you mentioned he had a history of with Dr. Peterson. That's consistent with prior exposure, but not particularly suggestive of current problems.

Kathleen : Okay.

Dr. Kaufman: His CBC, which is complete blood count, looks okay. His hematocrit blood count, which is the volume percentage of red blood cells, is a little high, and that actually could be from a little bit of dehydration.

Kathleen: Okay.

Dr. Kaufman: The next test is C. pneumoniae, which is a common form of pneumonia. It causes bacterial and upper respiratory infections, so we're all exposed to it, but usually we don't see the levels this high. So this may be quite relevant and something we need to talk about. Okay?

Kathleen: Okay.

Dr. Kaufman: I also checked his testosterone and thyroid levels because of his fatigue, and they're basically okay so that's not a problem. The next thing is his vitamin D level, which is extremely below normal, at twenty-four—not surprising since he doesn't go outside. We'd like to see that at about sixty to seventy, so we have to work on that. Then there's his arginine vasopressin.

Kathleen: Yeah?

Dr. Kaufman: That's a hormone produced by the pituitary gland. It's involved in helping maintain blood pressure by telling the kidneys to conserve fluid, and that test is extremely abnormal. Basically, it's undetectable. We see that very frequently in our patients with chronic fatigue syndrome. And it may partly explain why we can't elevate him.

Kathleen: Oh, okay.

Dr. Kaufman: Then there's his MTHFR mutation.

Me (thinking): *What the hell is that?*

Dr. Kaufman: This mutation, this gene, is involved in taking B12 and folic acid and converting them to their usable forms in the body. If they're not converted, we can't make use of them. They're vital, important vitamins for metabolic cycles related to energy, neurologic, and muscle function. The more mutations, the less able we are to convert, or methylate, those two vitamins.

Jamison is homozygous, meaning he has two mutations at the 677 site. There's two possible sites. This is a very significant mutation that may contribute to his illness, contribute to weakness, fatigue, and brain fog-type symptoms. He's had it since the moment he was conceived, so obviously people can live their whole lives having no problems with this mutation, but when they develop these neuro-immune, viral, immunologic diseases, the mutation adds to their problems. It's kind of like more snow on the snowball, or another domino, if you know what I mean. Now, I can't give him a new gene, but I can treat this with special vitamins. I'll come back to that. All right?

Kathleen: Sure.

Dr. Kaufman: Okay, so from the adrenal gland, do you know what cortisol is?

Kathleen: Yes.

Dr. Kaufman: Most of our patients have a dysfunction of what's called the hypothalamic pituitary axis, which, in the brain, sends signals to our endocrine organs. In this case, the dysfunction is in telling the adrenal glands when to make cortisol.

If you look at Jamison's day, his cortisol starts out at a little over five, instead of twenty-five. Then it continues to go down, and by evening he's totally below normal. This indicates either that his brain isn't properly instructing his adrenal glands about how much cortisol to produce, or it means that the adrenal gland itself is diseased and simply not able to follow instructions. Or it's both. The outcome is the same, which is a significant decrease, or lack of, cortisol and probably of a second hormone called aldosterone. The aldosterone is involved in maintaining blood pressure, so that may be why he's having trouble sitting upright. Cortisol is also a major hormone that helps deal with energy and stress.

Me (thinking): *That explains why you've felt so sick in stressful situations, and even enjoyable ones like having sex. You need cortisol to do these things.*

Dr Kaufman: As for the treatment, let me start with the easiest things. The vitamin D is D3. Any drugstore has it, and I'd like him to be on five thousand units a day.

Kathleen: Five thousand a day. Okay.

Dr. Kaufman: For the mutation that he has, he needs to be on what are called methyl-B12 and methyl-folate, so we bypass the impaired conversion by giving him pre-converted vitamins. The conversion takes B12 and makes it into methyl-B12. So I'm going to have him take methyl-B12 instead of the regular form. The methyl-folate will be a pill. Ultimately, I would like him on a fifteen-milligram pill.

Kathleen: Okay.

Dr. Kaufman: He takes that pill every day. Then, for methyl-B12, I would like to strongly urge that he takes the methyl-B12 as an injection, at least for the first month, three times a week. It's a very small needle. It's like taking a flu shot. Is that something you're going to be able to do?

Kathleen: Sure.

Dr. Kaufman: Many, many patients, particularly like Jamison, actually feel better almost in a matter of days with respect to some of their fatigue and brain fog when they start these vitamins. Now, let's see, do you have a blood pressure cuff there?

Kathleen: We do, yes.

Dr. Kaufman: Have you been measuring or have you ever measured his blood pressure and heart rate when he's in bed and then when he sits up?

Kathleen: We have. We were quite regular about it last spring, but lately it's been sporadic.

Dr. Kaufman: What kinds of readings have you gotten?

Kathleen: Let's see. I want to say . . . oh gosh, his heart rate was going above one hundred seventy. That might have been the highest lying flat.

Dr. Kaufman: Okay. What does he do now? Does he just lie flat in bed all the time?

Kathleen: Yes. All the time.

Dr. Kaufman: You can't raise the head of the bed forty-five degrees? He gets sick?

Kathleen: Yeah.

Dr. Kaufman: All right. I'm going to ask you to take some blood pressure and heart rate readings with the bed flat.

Kathleen: Sure.

Dr. Kaufman: And maybe thirty degrees instead of forty-five.

Kathleen: Okay.

Dr. Kaufman: You don't have to wait for him to get sick. You can just do it almost right away.

Kathleen: Okay, so you want us to do it flat first?

Dr. Kaufman: Flat and then as high as you can raise the bed without him really suffering. Do those readings and send them to me by email.

Kathleen: Will do.

Dr. Kaufman: All right. I'm going to talk to you about what I want to put him on and the results you send me may alter or adjust that, but because he's so sick, I don't want to wait to start treatment. Okay?

Kathleen: Yes.

Dr. Kaufman: Because the cortisol levels are so low, and because the other hormone is undetectable, we need to give him hormones to help his body manage his blood pressure better, and also cortisol for energy. Okay?

Kathleen: Okay.

Dr. Kaufman: I'm going to call in a prescription for hydrocortisone, which is what the adrenals produce. We're going to start him with ten milligrams in the morning. Usually people are on two or three doses. We're just going to start with one in the morning. Does he have a sleep-wake cycle? Does he wake up in the morning?

Kathleen: Yeah. He naturally wakes up for the day at maybe nine thirty, but often I will wake him up as I'm going to work before eight a.m.

Dr. Kaufman: Okay. When you go to work, is he alone in the house all day?

Kathleen: No. There's a caregiver here. She comes in about an hour after I leave.

Dr. Kaufman: What does he do during the day? I understand he's lying in bed, but does he watch television or anything?

Me (thinking): *Yeah, doc, it's Seinfeld reruns all day over here. No, come on, man. I'm in a dark cave. Caves don't have TVs.*

Kathleen: No, he's too ill to watch TV. Sometimes he's read to, though.

Dr. Kaufman: I see. Okay. We'll start with just the ten milligrams of hydrocortisone. It'll be a five milligram pill, so he'll take two.

Kathleen: Is that over the counter?

Dr. Kaufman: No. I'll have to call it in for you.

Kathleen: Great.

Dr. Kaufman: So, I'm going to do this sequentially. This is a little tricky for me, Kathleen, because I haven't even seen him. I hope you understand this is a little bit tricky. Okay. You and I are going to have to communicate a lot. Eventually, I'll want him on a higher dose, and I'll want him on a second hormone, but I'm going to do this in steps. After he's been on the ten milligrams for a few days, I'm going to ask you to tell me if you think it's helped him. And I'd like you to measure his blood pressure and heart rate again, just as you did to get his baseline.

Kathleen: Got it.

Dr. Kaufman: I'm going to ask you to give him an antibiotic for the C. pneumoniae, and that'll be a twice-a-day antibiotic. He's going to take that for ten days.

Kathleen: Okay.

Dr. Kaufman: Then lastly, we need to discuss an antiviral medication. You told me he was on Valtrex before. There are four antivirals: Famvir, Acyclovir, Valtrex, and Valcyte. So those first three, Acyclovir, Famvir, and Valtrex work against HH, HSV-1, HSV-2 and the Chickenpox virus. They don't work against CMV, and they don't usually work against Epstein-Barr. Valcyte is very effective against those. I think we actually should start him on the Valcyte, even though that's the most difficult drug to take. Often there are some side effects, and it requires some more monitoring. But I think that CMV is what's making him so sick.

Kathleen: Okay.

Dr. Kaufman: What's Jamison's insurance again?

Kathleen: It's a Medi-Cal insurance.

Dr. Kaufman: Then we may have trouble getting hold of the Valcyte. We're just going to have to try.

Kathleen: Okay.

Dr. Kaufman: Maybe if we're lucky, they'll approve it and cover it.

Kathleen: Potentially, I could put him on my insurance, but I don't really know that they would cover it either.

Dr. Kaufman: Well, let me explain the logistics of this. The FDA indication for Valcyte is for CMV. I can honestly and legitimately say he has an active CMV infection. If the insurance companies reject it, which they still often do, we can then turn to Genentech, the company that makes it. And if he has CMV, and if he lives in the US, and if he has an income below some number, and if he's been rejected by insurance, Genentech will pay for the drug and give it to us for free. But, there's one catch. If the patient has government insurance, Medicaid or Medicare, they often cannot do that. It's a quirk in the laws.

Kathleen: So, that's when I'd want to change his insurance?

Dr. Kaufman: Right. We can still—while he's on Medi-Cal—try to apply for it, but if he gets rejected, then you may need to consider changing his insurance.

Kathleen: Okay.

Dr. Kaufman: Kathleen, you need to be my eyes and ears because I can't see him, which means you shouldn't hesitate to contact me by email. I'm always going to want to know what you think has helped, or not helped, and what's happened. You might want to keep a little journal of medications and reactions and stuff.

Kathleen: Okay. I'll be keeping notes.

Dr. Kaufman: Good, I know there's a lot of stuff here. But I'm hoping that in a way it's good we have a lot of these things. There's some things I haven't been able to do because he's bed-bound, but we'll just work around that and figure it out as we go. Okay?

Kathleen: Okay, sounds good. Thank you!

* * *

I stop the recording, feeling even more optimistic about the treatments that Dr. Kaufman has prescribed for me. I was cynical, maybe even skeptical, after the first time I listened to the recording. But now that the treatments are working, I have much more confidence in Dr. Kaufman. He does make me wonder about the other doctors I've seen though. Had Dr. Gretchen and Dr. Peterson treated my illness differently, had they given me the medications that I'm currently on, I might not have gotten as sick as I am today. It just shows how much of my fate has rested in the hands of doctors, and how important it is to find the right one.

As I'm lying in bed, still thinking about the recording of Dr. Kaufman, the door to my room opens and my mom walks in.

"Hey, kiddo," she says. She sits down next to my bed. "How are you? Are you done listening to the recording?"

I smile and nod.

"Did you hear anything we missed?"

I shake my head.

"I should listen to it again. I will later. Right now it's just good to be with you," my mom says. I grab her hand, and she smiles at me. "I'm so glad I'm your mom. Jamison, you are such a strong person. It must be hard to hold on to who you are while you can't speak, but I will always know who you are. I cherish the person, the man, you've become."

I place my hand over my heart and start to tear up.

"And you know what? You *will* get better, and when you do, we are going on a cruise."

I hold up two fingers.

"Two? You need a bowel movement?" she asks.

I shake my head and try not to laugh. Then I make waves with my hand.

"Oh, you mean where are we going to take a cruise?" my mom asks, laughing. I smile and nod. "Oh, I don't know. How about the French Riviera?"

I give a thumbs up and look at her through my dark sunglasses. I can't remember the last time I was with my mom and didn't have something covering my eyes. So I take off the sunglasses, facing the harsh consequences of the bright sunlight coming in through the open door. The light stings my eyes, leaving a sort of carbon copy of the objects in the room stuck in my vision.

The pain eventually subsides, and my eyes focus on my mom's face. She's beautiful and tough. She's been through so much—working full-time and taking care of me, making sure I get the medical care that I need, among so many other logistical nightmares. She's been there for me through my darkest days. I truly believe that if I didn't have a strong will, she would have had enough for both of us. She wouldn't let me quit. And while there have been times of tension and frustration between us, the love we share has always prevailed. I want to tell her how grateful I am for everything that she's done for me—driving me to see doctors, buying and making me food, bathing me when I couldn't do it myself. The list of things my mom has done for me is as close to endless as it gets. And I know she feels my gratitude, but I'd still like to tell her, in my own way.

I point at myself, then put my hand over my heart, and finally point at her.

"Does that mean you love me?" she asks.

I put both of my thumbs up, then motion for her to come closer and I give her a kiss and a hug.

It's easy to remember all the things that I've lost—my voice, my muscles, my ability to walk—but my mom is a reminder of what I still have. Through it all, I've managed to hold on to the most important part of my life—the people I love. I can still hug and kiss my mom and my dad and Claire. And in this moment, that's all I need.

YEAR 7

A New Perspective

CHAPTER 54

Significantly Better

July 26, 2017

My mom was right when she said I would get better. I have gotten better. Significantly better. I can sit up in bed and tolerate more light coming in my room. On overcast days, and at dusk on sunny days, I open my drapes, which have replaced the thick blankets that used to cover my windows. And perhaps best of all, I can eat again. I'm limited to eating soft foods like avocado and pasta, but it's certainly better than having to drink liquified eggs through a straw. There have been few times in my life, if any, when I have experienced something, in this case chewing food again, that I've been deprived of for such an unimaginable amount of time. But I suppose where there has been deprivation, there is great joy to be found. There truly is no greater feeling, at least for me, than renewed experiences, and I've been having a lot of them lately.

I recently got out of bed on my own for the first time in more than two years. For several weeks, I had been gradually shifting my legs around and sitting on the edge of my bed without help. As I continued to get stronger, I eventually progressed to having my feet on the ground and trying to stand up on my own. That is when I encountered the greatest hurdle of all: pain.

When I tried to put my weight on my legs, my knees and ankles throbbed with inflammation. After so many months of being unable to stand up, my legs had become deconditioned. My muscles had atrophied, and my joints had grown rusty. But day after day, I kept at it, slowly putting more weight on my legs. Now I can stand upright and separate my body from the mattress that I've been on for so many months. I only last a few seconds before orthostatic intolerance makes my heart race and lungs burn, and I have to hold on to something to stabilize my balance, but the progress that I've made feels truly remarkable.

The treatments that Dr. Kaufman put me on—saline and vitamin infusions, B12 injections, an antiviral medication called Valcyte, and a steroid called hydrocortisone—have sustained my recovery. There have, however, been a few issues along the way. Paying for Dr. Kaufman's services has been expensive, often unaffordable. He charges more than five hundred dollars for a thirty-minute phone call, and he doesn't accept insurance, so my mom has had to ask friends and family to give me money to pay his bills. And then there's the difficulty of paying for, and subsequently taking, all of Dr. Kaufman's treatments. They cost thousands of dollars and make up a long list of medicines that I need to take each day, which hasn't always gone smoothly.

Because I'm still not well enough to travel to see Dr. Kaufman, and because he feels uncomfortable treating me remotely, he has transferred my prescriptions to a doctor near me. This way, the new doctor can monitor my progress more effectively. Working with yet another doctor and making sure he follows Dr. Kaufman's orders has been complicated at times, but I'm thankful for the medical care that I've received. So far, it seems to be working.

It's hard to pinpoint specifically which treatments are responsible for bringing me back to life because I started them all around the same time, but I would say the combination of hydrocortisone, Valcyte, and IV saline has helped me the most.

Taking Valcyte has improved my health by fighting the active viruses in my body, increasing my energy, and reducing my weakness. The hydrocortisone has come with some side effects—oily skin and a bloated face—but they're worth the benefits. The medication has helped me put weight on my shriveled body and raise my blood pressure. The saline has also improved my low blood pressure while hydrating my body and perfusing my kidneys, helping them to regulate my fluids and eliminate toxins. Saline infusions and hydrocortisone are the reason I'm now able to sit and stand on my own.

One thing I know from trial by error is that when I go several days without an infusion, I feel noticeably worse, and for some reason, I'm unable to adequately hydrate by drinking water and electrolytes. And there has been another significant discovery about my condition: Dr. Kaufman found that I have Lyme disease. The diagnosis was based on a positive antigen test and two coinfections. One of the infections is Borrelia, a type of bacteria associated with Lyme. The other is Babesia, a red blood cell parasite, which is also related to the disease. And it's all thanks to ticks.

I couldn't possibly have been bitten by a tick while I've been stuck in bed, which means I probably contracted the disease a long time ago—maybe as a kid playing in the Santa Cruz Mountains, or as a young adult hiking the foothills of Sonoma County. I do remember being bitten by a tick when I was in high school. I was doing a cardio workout on a baseball field wearing shorts. When I went to change my clothes, I noticed two dubious gray bugs attached to my calf. I was able to remove the ticks, and I went on with my life, but the moment now haunts me. Did I remove the ticks correctly? Were they attached long enough to transmit the disease? Were they even the kind of tick that carries Lyme disease?

Theoretically, the Lyme disease coinfections could have been festering in my body for a decade or longer. They could have remained latent, allowing me to go on with my normal life until a confluence of events occurred. Maybe the car accident damaged my brain and spinal cord, which compounded with my weakened immune system from overtraining for my bodybuilding competition. Then, along with Epstein-Barr and cytomegalovirus, Lyme disease could have activated, creating the perfect storm to take down a healthy, fitness-obsessed, college student in the prime of his life.

This, of course, is just one theory that may or may not prove to be true. Like my case of ME/CFS, there are many unknowns about my Lyme disease diagnosis. That's to say, I know more about my condition now than I have ever before, but I still know very little about it. And while I may never get answers to all of my questions, I don't plan to stop looking for them. For now, though, I'm content reaping the benefits of Dr. Kaufman's treatments.

One of the biggest benefits is that I've been able to move around more. The other day I went outside for the first time in two-and-a-half years. I slowly shuffled my body into a wheelchair, then my mom pushed me outside and, for a long time, I just sat on the deck and cried. There have been so many times when it seemed like I would never make it out of my room. I thought I'd be stuck in that tiny, dark space until I withered away and died. But sitting there on the deck, the fresh air hitting my face, I felt the most triumphant I've ever been in my life. I saw a view I had never seen before—the view outside my house. A gorgeous sunset lit up the vast Central Valley below me. The sprawling landscape stretched for dozens of miles, quite an improvement from looking at four walls and a ceiling all day.

My friend Thomas, who last saw me stuck in bed unable to do much of anything, was there to witness me emerge from the darkest days, and the darkest room, of my life. He looked so happy to see me doing better. As the sun went down, I tried to talk to Thomas just like when we were roommates back at Sonoma State. But my lungs weren't having it, and my jaw started hurting. To my relief, Thomas was content just taking in the view and enjoying the sunset. It was a marvelous sunset. The view gradually turned into a sliver of pink and purple sky, then disappeared below the horizon.

It was a once-in-a-lifetime moment. No, it was a never-in-a-lifetime moment. It was so special, and the circumstances so rare, that I feel bad for all the people who will never experience, or even imagine, how it felt. I laughed and cried and smiled. I couldn't have asked for a better way to transition out of the most horrific time in my life.

But as great as the moment was, I couldn't fully enjoy it—that I've had to transition at all feels like a blemish, as if the experience has been tainted. And the irony is that one wouldn't have existed without the other. I wouldn't have had such an incredible moment—a renewed experience after being deprived of fresh air and the setting sun—without being sick and having gone through hell first.

It's impossible not to feel tainted by the trauma of barely surviving for such a long time and the realization that nothing can replace the parts of my life that have been taken from me. But life goes on, and as it does, I may have to adjust my aspirations and find new goals to set my sights on, though only out of necessity and to curb mourning the parts of myself that may never again exist outside of my mind. The part of me that wants to be a bodybuilder will never die. The part of me that wants to find a soulmate to enjoy the rest of my life with will always remain in my heart.

These, and many other parts of me, will never fade and that is where I find my purpose and fulfillment. Regardless of what happens to me moving forward, I'm excited for the future. And it's been a long time since I've been able to say that.

CHAPTER 55

Shannon

December 8, 2017

Over the last several months, my health has mostly stayed the same, but I still have a lot to be hopeful about. I'm feeling better now than I have for most of the last three years. And there's a new development in my life—I'm in a relationship. My girlfriend, Shannon, who also has ME/CFS and Lyme disease, came into my world a few months ago and immediately gave me hope.

We met online, and after talking for a week, I told Shannon that I thought she was beautiful, both because I wanted her to know that I liked her, and because it was true—her piercing blue eyes and sweet smile stole my breath every time I looked at her avatar. She seemed unmoved by the gesture, though I'm not sure what I was hoping for, considering I couldn't see or hear her physical reaction. All I could see were the words she typed in response.

She thanked me graciously, but then the conversation ended. We didn't message each other for weeks, most likely because I thought my comment about her looks was too superficial or inappropriate. I also may have convinced myself that any sort of lasting affection from anyone I was attracted to was unrealistic at best. Sasha had given me affection when she crawled into bed with me and I kissed her, but I knew it was temporary, and so did she. After Sasha left, I came to expect that sort of fleeting love, if I expected it at all. But what I didn't know was that, unlike Sasha's, Shannon's affection wasn't on loan.

Luckily, a couple of weeks after our first interaction, she wished me happy birthday, and we became two friends with the same illness getting to know each other online—though there were also hints at a fledgling romance.

At one point I asked Shannon, "Do you think two sick people can be together?"

"Yes," she replied. "I think when you're both sick it makes it easier and harder at the same time."

"I guess the downside is there's no healthy person to take care of you," I said.

"But when you're alone, there's no healthy person to take care of you either," she replied.

I had never thought about it like that—the possibility of two sick people being in a successful relationship. I have always assumed that at least one person in a relationship would need to be healthy—two sick people can't take care of each other.

But I was wrong. Now that we're a couple, we take care of each other in ways I never imagined possible. I may not be able to make food for Shannon, but I can have takeout delivered to her. And she may not be able to be my caregiver, but she can post an ad looking for one. We've done these things and many others for each other, while she lives in Ontario, Canada, about two thousand miles from my house in California.

We support each other with an empathy that only two people with the same condition could feel. We know what the other person is going through on bad days; we know how exasperating it is to explain invisible symptoms to a doctor only to face skepticism. And all too well, we both know what it's like to be immobile creatures trapped in an ever-moving world.

Even so, we don't know everything about each other. We don't know what we were like as healthy people. We don't know what differences lie between our current selves and the people we were before getting sick and what maturation and emotional hardening has occurred during that transformation. But most fundamentally, we don't know what it's like to have a vocal conversation with each other.

Shannon has never heard my voice. She's never heard me berate a telemarketer or mumble to myself after making a typo. She's never heard me stumble through a dinner toast or tell a corny joke. She's never heard me whisper sweet nothings in her ear or come up with a witty retort. She's never heard me ask a question or speak my mind, to anyone. She may never get to hear me do these things, but that's okay. Here is this lovely woman, completely devoid of judgment, and she likes me for the unspoken words I type to her on a smartphone.

It's the first relationship I've had with what feels like real substance. I've finally found someone with whom I can share a romance, and at the same time, let my guard down without feeling shame. Shannon has an innate ability to disarm me, and in the process, she makes me feel as whole as possible, given the circumstances. We can't have sex and I can't lift weights, but through her, I feel more like the person I want to be than I ever have. Shannon contributes to this feeling not because I need someone to validate how I feel about myself, as I did before I got sick, but because she encourages my development as a whole person, instead of someone singularly focused on bodybuilding.

I have found someone whom I adore and who cares for me. In return, despite my weakened state, I make her feel loved. Ours has been anything but a conventional courtship. There's no precedent, no guidebook for our relationship, especially since our conditions are so unpredictable. I have no idea whether my health will continue to improve, or even remain stable, and I imagine Shannon feels similarly. For me, the thought of it no longer improving, or getting worse, absolutely terrifies me. Not a day goes by that I don't have this fear, and now that Shannon has infused my life with her presence, which I hold so dear, the fear has only elevated.

Every fear I have could materialize, or not. This time next year, Shannon and I could be driving down the California coast. Two years from now, we could be living together in Santa Cruz or maybe even Canada. Or maybe none of that will happen. We're both realistic and know there's the possibility, especially in our difficult situations, that things won't work out between us. But we're not focused on that. Right now we're just enjoying being together.

It's a special time for us because Christmas is coming, and we're together in person, not just messaging back and forth online. Shannon has had to travel across the continent to see me. And her willingness to do so, to jeopardize her health by traveling thousands of miles, makes me so grateful.

We are dreading her looming departure. We may not see each other again for months, maybe even years. But that's why we're determined to soak up the time. We have spent most of this week in bed, mostly holding each other, our bodies formed to one another like two pieces of a broken plate glued back together.

Because I still struggle to speak, we often communicate nonverbally. Most often, we resort to sending each other text messages while cuddling in bed. It's sort of like a month-long sleepover full of nonverbal communication. It's surreal—being stuck in a situation so miserable it could make your skin crawl while simultaneously finding comfort in knowing that someone you care about is right next to you, going through something similar.

But our experiences do differ. Shannon can briefly get up to use the bathroom, bathe, and on a good day, make herself a meal. I, on the other hand, still have to do everything in bed. Despite occasionally using my wheelchair to go outside and look at the sunset, I still have to bathe, urinate, and have bowel movements in bed. These are not sexy things, but they are part of life—my life and ours together.

I'll admit I was embarrassed, at least initially, to ask Shannon to look away and try not to think of me peeing mere inches from the spot in which we were kissing just seconds earlier. But I've since come to realize that it's all part of sharing our lives with each other. It may be far from the bedroom romps either of us had before getting sick, but knowing that nothing about my life makes Shannon uncomfortable endears her to me.

Perhaps that's why I have decided that now is the time to tell Shannon something that I've never told her before, something that has been on my mind since we first became a couple. I want to tell Shannon how much her companionship means to me because, among other things, she has given me the gift of affection and intimacy, two things that have been so vacant from my life.

Despite many previous attempts, I must tell her what I'm feeling. I've thought about just texting the words to her but that feels too inadequate, and using hand gestures feels far too clichéd. So I try to use my voice, and to my surprise, for the first time in months, I speak audibly.

Through a locked jaw and clinched teeth, I whisper, "I . . . love . . . you."

"What?" Shannon asks, seeming startled at the rarity of sound coming from my mouth.

I take a deep breath and fight back the nearly unbearable pain and weakness in my jaw, throat, and lungs. Tears well up in my eyes. Then, like so many times in the last several years, I feel a need to overcome, to do more, to keep going.

I whisper again, this time summoning all my strength: "I . . . love . . . you."

"Oh, sweetheart," Shannon says. "I'm so sorry. I don't know what you're saying." Then she takes my hand, gives me a soft kiss, and says, "You don't have to say anything . . . I love you."

EPILOGUE

The last time I saw Shannon, she visited me in California for ten days. Her mom came with her, and they spent some time in San Francisco before driving up to the Sierras to see me. For most of the visit, my mom hung out with Shannon's mom while we stayed in my room, snuggling. I still couldn't speak much, so Shannon did most of the talking and I texted her my responses.

Being with Shannon meant so much to me. Touching her soft skin after months of only virtual communication made me giddy, an endorphin rush that I never wanted to end. But it had to end. Shannon had to return to her life in Ontario, where her friends and family and obligations were waiting. I didn't want her to go. I wanted her to move to California and live with me, and for a brief time, it seemed like that was a possibility. But then Shannon got sicker. After she returned to Canada, her health drastically declined, and soon she was barely able to get out of bed and was almost never well enough to leave the house.

That was more than two years ago. Since then, things have been difficult for us. Shannon has continued to deal with a level of the illness that she has never experienced before, a severity that has at times made the future seem bleak and hopeless. And I've had my own challenges. My health hasn't gotten worse, but it hasn't exactly gotten better either. I'm still able to go outside in my wheelchair when I feel up to it, I can still enjoy the gastronomic pleasures of eating (lots of tacos and sandwiches), and I've even been able to speak audibly at times, but the plateau I've reached has made me wonder if there is a limit to my recovery. I had hoped to keep getting better, maybe even to be fully recovered by now.

It may have just been a quixotic fantasy, but I imagined myself recovering from the illness and flying to Canada to surprise Shannon. I had pictured a smile on her face when she opened the door and saw me walking and talking and doing everything a healthy person does. I had hoped to give her the biggest hug, maybe even use my renewed strength to pick her up and give her a million kisses all over her beautiful face as tears of joy ran down her cheeks. But that hasn't happened. Not yet, anyway.

Now that Shannon is sicker, and neither of us is well enough to travel, we're stuck two thousand miles apart on opposite sides of North America. We still talk every day, usually through text messages or on FaceTime. But, for everything we do to keep the relationship going, our future remains as uncertain as the probability that we'll see each other again.

We've both come to the conclusion that as much as we love each other and as important as it is for us to talk every day—to be each other's emotional support while battling a cruel illness—we can't have a complete relationship unless we're together in person. Until then, we're stuck in limbo, waiting for our health to improve, trying to hold on to the love we share.

That's why I'm afraid of losing Shannon. I'm scared that, after finding someone I connect with on such a deep level, I'll have to give her up because we're just too sick to be together. It feels selfish of me to take up so much of her time talking virtually when she could use that energy to find someone else, someone healthy who can be with her in person and care for her when she needs help. In the three years that I've known Shannon, too many times I've wanted to go over to her house and cook dinner for her or do her laundry, anything that would make her life easier while she's in the grips of the illness. It's been heartbreaking not to be able to do those things.

That's not to say that we don't take care of each other. We still do a lot for one another, as much as we can from afar. And that's why we're still so close, still such staples in each other's lives.

I don't know if my relationship with Shannon will last or, if it does, what shape it will take. But whatever happens, I'll always be thankful for Shannon. I met her at a scary time in my life, probably the scariest. My health was still unstable—I could barely eat, I couldn't speak, and I was living in constant fear of not being able to survive another day. To focus on my health, I had given up on many parts of a normal life, including finding love. Then one day, Shannon popped up on my phone and instantly made my life better. It was easy to fall in love with her, and in the process, she showed me so many things about myself and about being in a loving relationship.

Shannon has shown me that I can be in a relationship with someone I can't see in person. Though I talk to her every day, I rarely see her face, and even then, I only see it through the pixels on my phone. It's such a contrast to the relationships I've had in the past that were mostly based on physical attraction—my relationship with Molly was almost entirely about sex and working out, my relationship with Lily was a shotgun romance built on lust. The ironic part is that I'm more physically attracted to Shannon than I was to any of my previous girlfriends, but that's not why I love her. It doesn't hurt that she's stunningly gorgeous—her soft features and the way her mouth always seems to curl upward, even when she's not smiling, are absolutely adorable—but I love Shannon for other reasons. I love her for her sense of humor, for her easy-going nature, and for her empathy. She knows what I'm going through and, in turn, I understand her struggles. I try to reciprocate and give Shannon love and affection and empathy, but no matter how hard I try, I can't compete with her. As much as she makes me want to be a better person, I know she'll always be better than me in every way.

I talk to Shannon more than anyone else in the ME/CFS community, but I also keep in touch with others who have the disease, many of whom are just as sick as her. Some are even sicker and can't communicate, so I stay in contact with their caregivers. I've gotten to know Whitney Dafoe's mother, Janet, through texting and social media. Sometimes she calls me and, because I can't speak much, she just stays on the phone and gives me updates on how Whitney is doing and the progress that his father, Ron, continues to make in researching the illness.

I've never talked to Whitney, but through Janet I've learned how similar our stories are—we're around the same age and have spent years of our lives trapped in dark rooms. When I first got ME/CFS, I didn't know it was possible to be as debilitated as Whitney, but now I've experienced it, and it's still hard to imagine. The most baffling part is that there are likely millions of ME/CFS patients around the world who are just as sick—unable to walk, talk, or even eat—but no one knows about them because they're too sick to speak out, too sick to advocate for themselves.

The other day, I got a message from another friend with ME/CFS. Her condition had worsened, and she found herself too weak to get to the bathroom. As soon as I read her message, I got a sinking feeling because I knew what she was going through. Her fear was so palpable for me. I will never be able to forget the terror of realizing that I couldn't get to the bathroom. It's a primal fear, one that ignites an intense sense of desperation. Luckily we live in a time when there are solutions to these kinds of personal hygiene issues. I sent my friend links to buy a bedside urinal that drains into a sealed plastic bag on the ground and a commode that is basically a bucket with a raised seat. These things aren't fancy, and they can be messy, but they also make life better for those of us who can't get up to use the bathroom.

When I was first struggling with not being able to get to the bathroom, my family was compassionate and intuitive enough to help me get through it. My mom and Claire were able to put their heads together and figure out what I needed. It wasn't a pretty situation, or even a clean one, but we got through it. I'll always be indebted to my mom and Claire for that.

For a long time, Claire helped me in any way she could. She found people to take care of me while my mom was at work. She organized many of the parts of my life that I couldn't. But there were limits to how much she could help, and at times I got frustrated with my quality of life and took it out on her. She didn't deserve that. I feel bad that I wasn't more graceful in those moments, but thankfully Claire cut me slack and didn't take my unhappiness personally. Eventually she had to focus on her own life. She gave birth to my nephew, Dominic, and they now live in Alaska. We keep in touch through texting and FaceTime.

My dad also helped me get through the tough time, and he still supports me, but like Claire, he eventually returned home and focused on his own life.

Then, of course, there's my mom, who literally keeps me alive every day. She recently quit her job and now takes care of me full time. It's quite a juxtaposition to the early days of my illness, when I resisted her help at all costs. As my health deteriorated over the years, I had to adapt and let her do many vital tasks for me. I wouldn't have survived otherwise. I feel bad that I've essentially taken over my mom's life, but I'm also grateful that I get to spend each day with her.

Since my health has stabilized, and my mom has left her job, we've been able to settle into a more relaxed routine. She helps me for a few hours during the day and at night before she goes to bed. She brings me meals and helps me get into my inflatable bathtub, which goes on top of my mattress so I can bathe without having to move to the bathroom. I'm also able to do a lot of things for myself, like brush my teeth and shave. It feels good to become more self-sufficient, even though I'm far from as independent as I want to be.

I'm proud that I've made it this far, but because I'm still sick, it's easy for me to be cynical about my recovery—a reminder that some recoveries are more complete while others are more complex, and most aren't as they seem. Many people like to romanticize the recoveries of sick people because the mundane parts of our stories get overlooked and our most unflattering moments are easily omitted.

People leave out these parts of our stories because they don't fit the mold. They don't match the simple narrative that so often inspires people—someone got sick, then got better. I don't blame those who prefer that narrative. Shit, even I prefer that narrative. I love hearing about people who've had an illness or injury and, through sheer will and determination, brought themselves back to life. But it doesn't always work out like that. Lots of people get sick and never recover, and most who do get better don't have a linear recovery.

I'm an example of that. It's easy to tell people that I was sick and then got better. Everyone loves to hear that. It's inspiring. But it's not the whole story. The truth is much more complicated and difficult to explain. It's harder to describe how I got sick, then got a little better, then got sick again, then got so sick I almost died, then finally started to recover, only to plateau. Nobody latches on to that. It doesn't give anyone an abundance of hope. And it definitely doesn't fit into a neat little narrative. But it is the truth—my truth, my recovery.

AUTHOR'S NOTE

Some of the events I've written about in this memoir involve thoughts of suicide. If you are having similar thoughts, please reach out for help. You can call the National Suicide Prevention Lifeline at 800-273-8255.

While writing this book, I relied on my memory and various resources to recreate the events that took place in it. I used my personal journal and blog posts to begin a draft of the manuscript, then I consulted with people featured in the book to corroborate events and reconstruct dialogue, which may not always be verbatim. For many of the conversations with doctors and other medical professionals, I used audio recordings to reconstruct the dialogue; in one case, I had the audio professionally transcribed, then I edited it to fit within the book. In the case of the car accident, I referred to articles written about it, as well as the official accident report from the California Highway Patrol. And, because of my disabilities, I did it all on my smartphone.

For most of the book, with the exception of instances when I was too sick to write, I wrote a draft of the events shortly after they occurred, in some cases, mere minutes later. Writing in this form was very much a practice in contemporaneous note-taking, which is why the book is written predominantly in present tenses. While I did at times use past and future tenses, present tenses made the events more palpable and, having written in nearly real-time, I felt it was most natural and most accurate this way.

I changed nine names in the book—one doctor, one cat, and seven others. The rest of the names are real, as are all their identifying traits, though I did omit some for reasons of privacy. I also omitted some individuals who were peripherally involved but proved to be insignificant to the events that took place. Some of the dates and times are condensed and approximate, but as with all parts of the book, I tried to make them as accurate as possible.

Having said this, there are still bound to be mistakes within this book. It is not a flawless work. It is as imperfect as the person who wrote it. But it is my story to the best of my recollection.

ACKNOWLEDGMENTS

First, I want to thank my mom, Kathleen, who has supported me throughout my life and the writing of this book. Mom, thank you for everything you've done for me, for everything you continue to do each day, for keeping me going and getting me through some truly miserable times. It was more than anyone could handle, but somehow you handled it. I'll always be grateful for that, grateful for you.

My dad, Matt, has always supported me and encouraged me to finish this book. Dad, since I was a kid, you've treated me like a peer, an equal, a friend. I'm grateful that you've always been part of my life.

My sister, Claire, was also supportive along the way. Claire, I appreciate everything you've done for me. You have the biggest heart and the cutest son. I love you and Dom.

Shannon probably read this book more than anyone and helped me through more grammar questions than I care to count (or admit). Shannon, I'm so thankful that I met you. When we first started talking, I sent you an early draft of this book, and now you're in it. Thank you for letting me write about you, and about us. You have improved my life infinitely. I know we're still waiting for someone to lend us a jet so we can travel to see each other, but I'm happy that we're able to be together without, well, actually being together. Whether it's playing Animal Crossing or talking on FaceTime, we've managed to make an improbable virtual relationship work.

I want to thank Stephanie Land for writing the best foreword ever. Also a big thanks goes to Chelsea Page, Erica Verrillo, Kristen Hamilton, Kathleen Ortiz, and Linda Konner, all of whom helped me with this book in different ways at different times. I owe my gratitude to the tireless team at Inkshares for giving me the opportunity to publish the book. Avalon and Sarah, more than fifty publishers and at least a hundred literary agents rejected this book, but you agreed to put it out in the world, and I will never stop being thankful for that. I'm also appreciative of the incredible effort that Jocelyn Kelley has given to promoting the book.

I want to give a few shoutouts to insentient things. I want to thank technology for giving me the ability to write this book. Had smartphones not existed, I wouldn't have been able to write even half of these pages. The same goes for music, particularly songs by Jack Johnson, Adele, Johnnyswim, James Bay, and Sara Bareilles. When I was well enough to write, I was well enough to listen to music and boy did it help.

Lastly, I'm forever indebted to everyone who ordered this book and encouraged me to publish it. Thank you all!

ABOUT THE AUTHOR

A former Christmas tree salesman, Jamison graduated from Sonoma State University and has gone on to write for *The New York Times*, the *Washington Post, Men's Journal,* the *Los Angeles Times*, and *Writer's Digest*, among other publications. Jamison has been a guest on Dax Shepard's *Armchair Expert* podcast and was featured in a Netflix original series. Jamison's *New York Times* essay, "Love Means Never Having to say . . . Anything," was adapted for WBUR's *Modern Love* podcast and read by Pedro Pascal (*The Mandalorian*). You can follow Jamison on Instagram (@NotLikeTheWhiskey), Twitter (@ NotTheWhiskey), and his blog (JamisonWrites.com).

GRAND PATRONS

Adrian Godby
Aleasha Ross
Amanda L. Williams
Amy Mooney
Ann Mc Donald
Beth Mc Clelland
Chad H. Black
Cindy Siegel Shepler
Dana Rieger
Dawn M. Rodrigues
Elizabeth W. Friedrich
Heather Dreske
Jacqueline Naiditch
Jane Pannell
Janet Edmonds Barrella
Jen Taylor
Karen M. Scott
Kathe Hilberman & Michael Lasky
Kevin Rice & Kathy Tellin

Liz Burlingame
Mary T. Danze
Marcia Sanchez
Mary de Rosas
Maureen O'Halloran
Morgan Roth
N. Dreske
Patricia J. Hill
Ryan O. Toole
Sandee Whalen
Shannon Donegan
Solona Armstrong
Suzanne Jennings
Tammy Pennington
Tilman Andris
Tommy Stribling
Tom Yeung
Traci Lynn Bumpus

INKSHARES

INKSHARES is a reader-driven publisher and producer based in Oakland, California. Our books are selected not by a group of editors, but by readers worldwide.

While we've published books by established writers like *Big Fish* author Daniel Wallace and *Star Wars: Rogue One* scribe Gary Whitta, our aim remains surfacing and developing the new author voices of tomorrow.

Previously unknown Inkshares authors have received starred reviews and been featured in the *New York Times*. Their books are on the front tables of Barnes & Noble and hundreds of independents nationwide, and many have been licensed by publishers in other major markets. They are also being adapted by Oscar-winning screenwriters at the biggest studios and networks.

Interested in making your own story a reality? Visit Inkshares.com to start your own project or find other great books.